Communication and Interpersonal Skills for Nurses

Series Editor: Shirley Bach

Transforming Nursing Practice – titles in the series

To order, contact our distributor: BEBC Distribution, Albion Close, Parkstone, Poole, BH12 3LL. Telephone 0845 230 9000, email: **learningmatters@bebc.co.uk**. You can also find more information on each of these titles and our other learning resources at **www.learningmatters.co.uk**

Communication and Interpersonal Skills for Nurses

Shirley Bach and Alec Grant

First published in 2009 by Learning Matters Ltd

British Library Cataloguing in Publication Data
A CIP record for this book is available from the British Library

ISBN: 978 1 844 451 623

Cover design by Toucan Design
Project Management by Diana Chambers
Typeset by Kelly Gray
Printed and bound in Great Britain by TJ International Ltd, Padstow, Cornwall

Learning Matters Ltd
33 Southernhay East
Exeter EX1 1NX
Tel: 01392 215560
E-mail: info@learningmatters.co.uk
www.learningmatters.co.uk

Contents

Foreword

As someone who supports students in clinical placements, I am struck by how often it is the subtle intricacies around how we communicate and interact with patients, families and colleagues that present us as nurses with the greatest intellectual and emotional challenges. Numerous dilemmas, confusions, misunderstandings and anxieties arise as we try to tease out what we bring to the game as individuals, what we encounter in our roles as students and nurses, and what are complex aspects of the patients, relatives, professionals and organisations we engage with.

It is in this light that I welcome this excellent book, in which the authors span a breadth of interesting, pertinent and at times refreshing array of topics that are important in considering communication and interpersonal skills in all fields of nursing. In places, rather demanding concepts are explored, but it is worth the effort as the authors illuminate nursing practice by drawing on core evidence from nursing and then venture outside the traditional stomping ground to pull in research, theories and ideas belonging to other fields. This lateral approach promises to stimulate nursing students and others to explore how best to make sense of the complexities and challenges of communication and interpersonal relationships.

The book looks at some of the typical stumbling blocks many of us encounter as we strive to learn how to communicate and interact safely and effectively, and offers ways to anticipate and engage with the potential barriers that often lead to emotional struggles for students in practice. Practical can-do exercises within these pages offer students scope to reflect on their personal and clinical experiences and relate these to the focus of a particular chapter. Many of these interactive elements could prove to be prize material in class-based teaching and learning.

The chapter on the learning and educational context should be valuable to many students and mentors as it provides a wholesale exploration of how the student experience, both in university and practice, fits within a broader educational framework. The results of engaging with this should be a more empowered student who takes greater ownership of their education and mentors that can better appreciate how the sum of the parts fits together.

The last two chapters shed a bright light on the social-cultural settings within which nursing practice, interpersonal interactions and communication take place. These rich, thoughtful and wide-ranging sections scrutinise the challenges of providing effective healthcare across the lifespan within a constantly evolving, diverse society.

I came away from reading this book with new concepts and understanding that will inform my work with students and qualified nurses for years to come. It is with great pleasure that I commend it to you.

Dr Alan Simpson
Senior Research Fellow and Lecturer
Vice-Chair, Mental Health Nurse Academics (UK)
City University, London

Acknowledgements

The authors and publisher would like to thank the following for permission to reproduce copyright material:

Arnold, E and Boggs, KU, *Interpersonal Relationships: Professional communication skills for nurses*. Copyright © 2006, Elsevier, London.
Adapted Table 5.1, 'Comparison of social and professional relationships', p77, reproduced with kind permission of Elsevier, London.

Dai, DY and Sternberg, RJ (eds) *Motivation, Emotion and Cognition*. Copyright © 2004, Lawrence Erlbaum, Mahwah, NJ.
Adapted Theory Summary, p89, reproduced with kind permission of Lawrence Erlbaum, Mahwah, NJ.

DeVito, JA, *The Interpersonal Communication Book*. Copyright © 2007, Pearson Education Inc., Upper Saddle River, NJ.
Adapted table in Activity 5.3, p85, and Relationships and proxemic distances box, p82, reproduced with kind permission of Pearson Education Inc., Upper Saddle River, NJ.

Hargie, O and Dickson, D, *Skilled Interpersonal Communication. Research, Theory and Practice*. Copyright © 2004, Routledge, London and New York.
Adapted Types of Self box, p84, reproduced with kind permission of Routledge, London and New York.

Kreps, G and Kunimoto, EN, *Effective Communication in Multicultural Health Care Settings*. Copyright © 1994, Sage Publications, London.
Adapted Figure 8.1 'Iceberg model of multicultural influences on communication', p149, reproduced with kind permission of Sage Publications, London.

Narayanasamy, A, The ACCESS model: a transcultural nursing practice framework. *British Journal of Nursing*, 11(9): 643–50. Copyright © 2002, *British Journal of Nursing*. The ACCESS model, p154, reproduced with kind permission of the *British Journal of Nursing*.

Rose, D and Pevalin, DJ (2005) *The National Statistics Socio-economic Classification: Origins, development and use*. Institute for Social and Economic Research, University of Essex. Basingstoke: Palgrave Macmillan. Crown copyright © 2005.

'Social class based on occupation', p156, 'Socio-economic groups', p157 and 'Operative categories of the National Statistics socio-economic classification (NS-SEC)', p158. Reproduced under the terms of the Click-Use License.

Every effort has been made to trace all copyright holders within the book, but if any have been inadvertently overlooked the publisher will be pleased to make the necessary arrangements at the first opportunity.

About the authors

Dr Shirley Bach is Head of the School of Nursing and Midwifery at the University of Brighton and also the Series Editor for *Transforming Nursing Practice*. In the past, she designed curricula for nurses that integrated interpersonal relationship skills and communication studies, before specialising in health psychology and the application of psychology to health and illness settings. She has written a study guide in psychology for nurses, and researched and developed a model for psychological care. She has also led programmes that promote the professional practice of nursing and midwifery, especially in the area of advanced nursing practice. Most recently, she has developed an interest in new learning technologies and has drawn upon her understanding of both communication and pedagogic theories to publish in this area.

Dr Alec Grant is Principal Lecturer in the School of Nursing and Midwifery at the University of Brighton and is a Registered and Accredited Cognitive Psychotherapist. With a background in, originally, mental health nursing, and more latterly psychotherapy, social science and psychology, he is now a course leader for the M.Sc. in Cognitive Behavioural Psychotherapy. He has taught, researched, practised and written about communication and interpersonal skills – and related areas such as clinical supervision – in the caring profession since the mid-1970s.

Introduction

Who is this book for?

This book is primarily intended for students of nursing, whether on a diploma or degree pathway, starting their Common Foundation Programme or equivalent. However, as communication and interpersonal skills (CIPS) develop throughout the course as different contexts and situations are faced, the relevance of the topic will still apply in years two and three. The focus is not to develop knowledge for any one specific branch (Adult, Child, Mental Health or Learning Disabilities) but to support development for progress into any branch and beyond. Therefore, there may well be value for those who are studying on branch programmes and those on continuing professional development modules. It may also be of interest to experienced nurses who wish to develop their leadership roles. The Nursing and Midwifery Council's (NMC) *Standards of Proficiency for Pre-registration Nursing Education* are a foundation for the book. However, the content is not narrowly defined by them.

Why communication and interpersonal skills for nursing?

Because we have learned since birth how to express ourselves within our family and friendship groups, we all believe we are good at communicating. We have also been honing our relationship skills, often through trial and error or role modelling, and we think there is no need to consider very deeply about how we do it. It has become second nature. There are times, though, when we experience situations where we consider that an interaction did not go smoothly; perhaps we were misunderstood or a friend reacted differently to how we expected. At times like these, we may think that we could have said something differently that would have improved the reactions and responses of ourselves and those around us. So, while we have developed expertise, we can always learn and improve when it comes to human relationships, mainly because there are so many factors that influence how we respond in various situations.

If we shine the spotlight on healthcare situations, where there are many complexities that are often similar to our everyday lives but enhanced by factors such as healthcare policy, environment, hierarchies of responsibility, physical discomfort, anxiety, sadness and fear, we have an even more complicated set of circumstances to deal with than when we communicate or interact with family or friends. Healthcare interactions are with patients, carers and peers in often demanding and stressful circumstances, which inevitably lead to further demands on our abilities to communicate effectively. Therefore, it is important that students take time to learn in more detail about communicating in healthcare settings in order to interact as effectively as possible. This means becoming more aware of oneself as well as others.

Unfortunately, there is ample literature to suggest that we do not communicate as well as we might in healthcare settings. In this book we will be exploring the many factors that impact on our abilities to communicate ideas to one another in these settings. We will try to rise to the challenge of improving CIPS interactions in our different spheres of practice.

Learning features

We will draw on evidence from the nursing literature, theories of nursing, social psychology, sociology, communication studies and contemporary issues for twenty-first-century living to provide you with insights on improving your CIPS. There will be activities to engage you with the ideas by utilising self-assessments, case studies and scenarios. Some of these will be activities you undertake as self-reflection, while others may involve discussion with your fellow students. There will also be practical activities and references to further reading or websites for you to explore. We have included a glossary of some terms that we also hope will help explain ideas and concepts covered in the chapters (glossary terms are bold in the text).

Book structure

In Chapter 1, 'Nursing, caring and interpersonal communication', we introduce the subject and examine the issues facing today's nurses in achieving effective and safe CIPS. We explore the fundamental concepts of communication and of interpersonal skills and differentiate between the two. This is done through the lens of the caring domain of nursing as a context for improving CIPS. The final section of the chapter describes a systematic framework for CIPS in nursing.

In Chapter 2, 'Key concepts', the crucial need for effective and sophisticated interpersonal communication in modern healthcare organisations is discussed. The key concepts in CIPS are defined, and explained, together with the underpinning theories. This discussion will help students to understand and justify why good interpersonal communication makes a significant difference to nursing practice. The chapter differentiates between CIPS in nursing and in counselling and psychotherapy. The case for an evidence base for CIPS in nursing is outlined and the nursing, and related, theories underpinning interpersonal communication in nursing are explored. Finally, the organisational basis for healthy interpersonal relating in nursing is discussed.

In Chapter 3, 'Evidence-based principles', we explore key issues in the historical development of research in CIPS in nursing. The effectiveness of research into CIPS teaching and experiential learning is discussed. The chapter articulates the problems around a sole reliance on humanistic counselling/psychotherapy models of communication. We evaluate the reasons for the importance of good interpersonal and organisational climates in the practice of nursing CIPS. Patient/client first- and second-level forms of communication are explored to provide a deeper understanding. The meaning behind 'blip cultures' and the forms of communication appropriate to such cultures is considered in relation to evidence-based practice.

Chapter 4, 'Safe and effective practice', aims to increase understanding of the importance and relevance of a process for communicating safely and effectively. The hidden areas of interpersonal communication are explored to enable practice in a safe manner, with examples of techniques to draw upon. The many roles that are embedded in CIPS and the healthcare context are examined to enable clarity and effectiveness. Strategies to identify and describe techniques to develop an effective communication relationship process are explained and models for helping relationships are described and compared before being applied to healthcare situations.

In Chapter 5, 'Understanding potential barriers', we explore the underpinning reasons for barriers to communication and describe techniques to resolve the barriers. We begin by distinguishing between social and professional relationships and the rules of social engagement. The relevance of emotions in communication and the need to balance emotions in effective interpersonal relationships are explored. The impacts of interpreted meanings, motivation for health and conflict, as barriers to communication in healthcare, are explored with suggestions and practical techniques for overcoming difficult situations.

Chapter 6, 'The learning and educational context', takes a different perspective on CIPS by exploring how classroom theory and practice can be integrated by understanding how skills can be learned. We discuss the theory underpinning learning from experience so that learning can be based on reality. So that students can understand what is expected at different academic levels, we examine the different levels of learning that are expected in students' assessed work. We take time to explore how reflection can be effectively managed in portfolios for the assessment of practical skills. Different activities are identified that will enhance communication in learning and teaching situations. The chapter closes with an exploration of the principles of lifelong learning – based on the premise that we never stop learning and improving our knowledge and skills if we strive to be knowledgeable and competent practitioners.

We begin Chapter 7, 'The environmental context', by exploring the broader aspects of the impact of environment on CIPS and how different care settings might undermine safe and effective practice. The impact of physical and social environmental factors on the practice of good communication in healthcare is considered and examples of each are given with groups or families and younger and older people. 'Prejudice' and 'schema development' and their relation to language use in nursing are explored. The chapter aims to enhance appreciation of the demands on CIPS in British nursing caused by the nature of multiculturalism as an environmental construct. The impact of institutional racism on CIPS in British nursing practice and healthcare organisations is also discussed. The meaning of the 'fallacy of individualism' as it pertains to CIPS in nursing care is explored and the responsibility of the organisation and the individual in CIPS.

Finally, Chapter 8, 'Population and diversity contexts', takes a look at the impact of our contemporary society on CIPS by examining diversity from different perspectives. We begin by considering the needs and diversity of populations and the individuals within them. Our first approach to this is to recognise that care must be respectful and anti-discriminatory and that there is a need for equity and fairness. Defining culture and exploring theories underpinning approaches to CIPS in culturally varied populations is a key aspect of this section in the chapter. We go on to examine diverse groups in society, such as socio-economic position, race and culture, gender, sexual orientation, age and disability. We conclude by exploring ethical and moral issues in communicating with diverse groups in healthcare settings.

Requirements for the NMC *Standards of Proficiency*

The NMC (2004a) has published standards to be achieved by all students in their first year before they can progress to the Branch Programme. These standards are to be used by the educational organisations when planning and designing their courses. For entry to the branch, the domains that are used to guide the content of this book are Professional and ethical practice, Care delivery, Personal and professional development and Care management. They are outlined in the following table.

NMC STANDARD 7 – FIRST LEVEL NURSES – NURSING STANDARDS OF EDUCATION TO ACHIEVE THE NMC STANDARDS OF PROFICIENCY

DOMAIN: PROFESSIONAL AND ETHICAL PRACTICE

Manage oneself, one's practice and that of others in accordance with *The NMC Professional Code of Conduct, Performance and Ethics*, recognising one's own abilities and limitations

Outcomes to be achieved for entry to the branch programme

Demonstrate an awareness of The NMC Code of Professional Conduct: Standards for conduct, performance and ethics

Practise in accordance with an ethical and legal framework which ensures the primacy of patient and client interest and well-being and respects confidentiality

Outcomes to be achieved for entry to the branch programme

Demonstrate an awareness of, and apply ethical principles to, nursing practice

- demonstrate respect for patient and client confidentiality
- identify ethical issues in day to day practice.

Practise in a fair and anti-discriminatory way, acknowledging the differences in beliefs and cultural practices of different individuals and groups

Outcomes to be achieved for entry to the branch programme

Demonstrate the importance of promoting equity in patient and client care by contributing to nursing care in a fair and anti-discriminatory way

- demonstrate fairness and sensitivity when responding to patients, clients and groups from diverse circumstances

---

- recognise the needs of patients and clients whose lives are affected by disability, however manifest.

DOMAIN: CARE DELIVERY

Engage in, develop and disengage from therapeutic relationships through the use of appropriate communication and interpersonal skills

Outcomes to be achieved for entry to the branch programme

Discuss methods of, barriers to, and the boundaries of, effective communication and interpersonal relationships

- recognise the effect of one's own values on interactions with patients and clients and their carers, families and friends
- utilise appropriate communication skills with patients and clients
- acknowledge the boundaries of a professional caring relationship.

Demonstrate sensitivity when interacting with and providing information to patients and clients.

Create and utilise opportunities to promote the health and well-being of patients, clients and groups

Outcomes to be achieved for entry to the branch programme

Contribute to enhancing the health and social well-being of patients and clients by understanding how, under the supervision of a registered practitioner, to:

- contribute to the assessment of health needs
- identify opportunities for health promotion.

Undertake and document a comprehensive, systematic and accurate nursing assessment of the physical, psychological, social and spiritual needs of patients, clients and communities

Outcomes to be achieved for entry to the branch programme

Contribute to the development and documentation of nursing assessments by participating in comprehensive and systematic nursing assessment of the physical, psychological, social and spiritual needs of patients and clients

- be aware of assessment strategies to guide the collection of data for assessing patients and clients and use assessment tools under guidance
- discuss the prioritisation of care needs
- be aware of the need to reassess patients and clients as to their needs for nursing care.

Formulate and document a plan of nursing care, where possible, in partnership with patients, clients, their carers and family and friends, within a framework of informed consent

Outcomes to be achieved for entry to the branch programme

Contribute to the planning of nursing care, involving patients and clients and, where possible, their carers; demonstrating an understanding of helping patients and clients to make informed decisions

- identify care needs based on the assessment of a patient or client
- participate in the negotiation and agreement of the care plan with the patient or client and with their carer, family or friends, as appropriate, under the supervision of a registered nurse
- inform patients and clients about intended nursing actions, respecting their right to participate in decisions about their care.

Based on the best available evidence, apply knowledge and an appropriate repertoire of skills indicative of safe and effective nursing practice

Outcomes to be achieved for entry to the branch programme

Contribute to the implementation of a programme of nursing care, designed and supervised by registered practitioners

- undertake activities that are consistent with the care plan and within the limits of one's own abilities.

Demonstrate evidence of a developing knowledge base which underpins safe and effective nursing practice

- access and discuss research and other evidence in nursing and related disciplines
- identify examples of the use of evidence in planned nursing interventions.

Demonstrate a range of essential nursing skills, under the supervision of a registered nurse, to meet individuals' needs, which include:

- maintaining dignity, privacy and confidentiality; effective communication and observational skills, including listening.

Domain: Care management

Contribute to public protection by creating and maintaining a safe environment of care through the use of quality assurance and risk management strategies

Outcomes to be achieved for entry to the branch programme

Contribute to the identification of actual and potential risks to patients, clients and their carers, to oneself and to others, and participate in measures to promote and ensure health and safety

- understand and implement health and safety principles and policies
- recognise and report situations that are potentially unsafe for patients, clients, oneself and others.

Demonstrate knowledge of effective interprofessional working practices which respect and utilise the contributions of members of the health and social care team

Outcomes to be achieved for entry to the branch programme

Demonstrate an understanding of the role of others by participating in interprofessional working practice

- identify the roles of the members of the health and social care team
- work within the health and social care team to maintain and enhance integrated care.

DOMAIN: PERSONAL AND PROFESSIONAL DEVELOPMENT

Demonstrate a commitment to the need for continuing professional development and personal supervision activities in order to enhance knowledge, skills, values and attitudes needed for safe and effective nursing practice

Outcomes to be achieved for entry to the branch programme

Demonstrate responsibility for one's own learning through the development of a portfolio of practice and recognise when further learning is required

- identify specific learning needs and objectives
- begin to engage with, and interpret, the evidence base which underpins nursing practice.

Acknowledge the importance of seeking supervision to develop safe and effective nursing practice

NMC *Essential Skills Clusters*

In addition to the *Standards of Proficiency*, the NMC (2007) has published essential skills that students have to achieve before entry into their chosen branch and for registration. These provide detailed, baseline skills descriptors for fundamental care. The two clusters that are covered in this book are:

1. Care compassion and communication, and
2. Organisational aspects of care.

Readers are encouraged to access these skills clusters to inform their practice assessments.

1. Nursing, caring and interpersonal communication

CHAPTER AIMS

After reading this chapter, you will be able to:

- understand the issues facing nursing today in achieving effective and safe communication and interpersonal skills (CIPS);

- explore the concepts of CIPS and differentiate between the two;

- explore the caring domain of nursing as a context for improving CIPS;

- describe a systematic framework for CIPS in nursing.

Introduction

From very early times, when *Homo sapiens* began to evolve and cohabit in an environment that was both hostile and primitive, one of the first skills it was imperative to learn was the **communication** of ideas. This enabled the men and women of those times to share understandings, protect one another and develop new ideas to solve the problems they encountered in their everyday lives – in order to survive. We can also hazard a guess that, after a while, they were not only communicating facts about where to find the best berries or tracks of the nearest herd of woolly mammoths. Could they have shared a joke, or expressed rage, excitement, fear, desire or jealousy? Would they have sighed in mutual appreciation over a beautiful sunset or puzzled over the origins of shooting stars? Could they have pointed out the best and worst places to hunt or the value of one animal fur garment over another? If they did, they would have added to their repertoire of communication skills certain enhancements to elaborate concepts that could not be drawn in the earth with a stick or painted on a cave wall.

So that communication between each other could be more easily understood by early *Homo sapiens*, different modes of communication were developed. Anthropologists tell us that they believe drawing was the first means of meta-communication. Over time, language was developed and refined from sounds to form commonly understood words and phrases. Methods of communication for language in the written and spoken form have continued to evolve over the millennia to the extent that, in our present world, we are using highly technological methods such as the internet and other electronic formats.

These enhancements, due to the kinship groups and social networks evidenced by anthropological evidence, would have developed from, and been based around, the connectedness of the individuals and their relationships. These basic premises have not changed for us in our current day-to-day activities. The means of communication may have advanced and become more varied and technical, but the basic human need to communicate and share ideas with those we know, work with or care for has not changed.

In this chapter we will begin by exploring the issues that face nursing today and the need for safe and effective communication and **interpersonal skills** (CIPS). We will then begin to explore the concepts of CIPS. Chapter 2 will expand on several key concepts that combine to shape collectively our communication and interpersonal activities. This chapter goes on to discuss the caring domain of nursing as a guiding principle for establishing relational aspects of nurse–patient encounters.

In the subsequent chapters in this book you will find guidance, theories, explanations and activities on how to improve your communication and interpersonal understanding and skills. In this chapter we will outline how you can begin to put this information into a generic and systematic framework to assess situations, plan, make decisions, review and end communication and interpersonal interactions.

Issues facing nursing today

The World Health Organization (WHO) (2000), European Union (EU) (2004), Department of Health (DH) (2004) and the National Health Service (NHS) Modernisation Agency (2003) have all emphasised the importance of patient-focused communication between health professionals and patients. This is seen as vital to achieving patient satisfaction, inclusive decision making in caregiving and an efficient health service. Nursing literature also promotes these concepts as indicative of best practice (for example, McCabe and Timmins, 2006 and NMC, 2004b). Charlton et al. (2008) found that, by using a person-centred approach in the interaction between nurses and patients, care outcomes were improved in:

- patient satisfaction;
- adherence to treatment options;
- patient health.

However, there is some evidence to suggest that, while qualified nurses often rate their own communication skills as high, patients report less satisfaction and maintain that communication could be improved. In addition, there is evidence that some nurses stereotype patient groups (Timmins, 2007).

There are criticisms of teaching CIPS in nursing education that point to a lack of systematic evaluation of teaching and a difficulty in resolving the difference between the *school way and the ward way* (Chant et al., 2002). There is a need to consider learning these skills in the clinical environment with greater involvement of clinical staff. The aim of this book is to contribute to the learning of CIPS, to give students an opportunity to think about their own CIPS and to seek opportunities to practise achieving their CIPS learning outcomes in the practice environment.

Effective communication is also essential to practice and improving interpersonal relationships in the workplace between professional groups and peers

(Grover, 2005). It is acknowledged that successful communication is shaped by basic techniques, such as open-ended questions, listening, **empathy** and assertiveness. However, successful interpersonal relationships are also affected by intervening variables, such as professional ideologies, gender, generation, context, collegiality, cooperation, self-disclosure and reciprocity, which can impede or enhance the outcome of quality communication.

The more recent emphasis on dignity and respect from the DH, and the professional bodies such as the Royal College of Nursing (RCN) and NMC, has highlighted the issues for sections of the public that have not received quality care from health professionals. The Dignity in Care Campaign (**www.dh.gov.uk/en/SocialCare/Social carereform/Dignityincare/DH_6600**) aims to end tolerance of indignity in health and social care services through raising awareness and inspiring people to take action. Older people and persons with mental health and/or learning disabilities have been highlighted as care groups that require special attention in healthcare services for personalised care. The role of person-centred care and CIPS is integral to the accommodation of these care groups.

In a similar vein 'The Essence of Care' series has been designed by the DH to support the measures to improve quality, and will contribute to the introduction of clinical governance at local levels (**www.dh.gov.uk/en/Publicationsandstatistics/ publications/PublicationsPolicyAndGuidance/DH_4005475**). The benchmarking process outlined in the 'Essence of Care' helps practitioners to take a structured approach to sharing and comparing practice, enabling them to identify the best and to develop action plans to remedy poor practice. Essence of Care guidelines have been produced for clinical governance, promoting health and the care environment.

ACTIVITY 1.1   REFLECTIVE

Recall a care setting that you have visited recently and think about the levels of dignity and respect given to the patients in that setting. Would you consider that there needs to be improvement? If yes, visit the website of the DH where the 'Essence of Care' audit tools are located and download a tool that relates to a situation you have experienced in practice. Identify where you would improve the care in that environment, if you were a member of the healthcare team.

As this activity is based on your own reflection, there is no outline answer at the end of the chapter.

In 2007, the NMC published the *Essential Skills Clusters*, which include 'Care, Compassion and Communication (NMC, 2007). The skills are to be used in conjunction with the NMC *Standards of Proficiency* in all pre-registration courses from 2008, with sets of skills to be achieved prior to entry to branch and to the register. The first three skills that are relevant to entry to branch are highly relevant to this discussion and exemplify the importance of communication with care, dignity and respect. They are shown in the following box.

ACTIVITY 1.2   REFLECTIVE

Reflect on the essential skills that are listed under Care, Compassion and Communication. Download a copy of the skills, if you do not already have a copy, and think about how you will improve your care in relation to these skills. Against each of the skills from 1 to 3 make a note of every time you see a qualified nurse carry out care that reflects these skills and note for yourself how they do this, how you could adopt best practice in this skill and how you will carry out these skills in the future to achieve a high, professional standard of care.

What do you think prevents these essential skills being carried out and how do you think these 'blocks' can be improved?

As this activity is based on your own reflection, there is no outline answer at the end of the chapter.

Fundamental concepts in communication and interpersonal skills

We might think that, straightaway, we know how the concepts of 'communication' and 'interpersonal skills' can be described and the meaning associated with the terms – and can sum this up in one sentence. OK, you have a go!

ACTIVITY 1.3   PRACTICAL

In one sentence, describe what communication is and means without looking in a dictionary!

In another sentence, sum up what interpersonal means.

_____

As this activity is based on your own reflection, there is no outline answer at the end of the chapter.

Check out your sentences with the following definitions:

Communication is to exchange information between people by means of speaking, writing or using a common system of signs or behaviour.

Interpersonal describes the connection between two or more people or groups and their involvement with one another, especially as regards the way they behave towards and feel about one another.

How close were you to the definitions supplied by Encarta?

THEORY SUMMARY

What is a concept?

In general, it is accepted that a concept is a broad theoretical idea that someone has thought up, or named, to help us picture how an intangible idea can be understood and to enable us to express this idea through language. To take this discussion one step further, concepts are also deemed to be abstract, that is, not concrete, but expressing a quality, emotion or thought, and thus something you cannot necessarily see or touch. A concept can also be deemed a principle that guides somebody's actions, especially one that has a value or importance attached to the ideas, to be followed as a guide for human behaviours and responses. Exploring concepts is a means of describing and analysing incidents, and a technique used extensively in this book, to capture the meaning of how, for example, people behave, or how nature, reality or events are perceived.

It would be helpful to consider the difference between the two concepts of communication and interpersonal skills and why we have brought them together in this book. Exchanging information through the communication of ideas, fact and emotions is a complex phenomenon, and cannot take place in nursing without the recognition of the many context-specific factors that influence the communication. Communication, as you will discover in subsequent chapters, requires many different methods and processes to become effective. Even when we are not communicating, invoking silence for example, we are communicating a message with a meaning that will need to be interpreted. Consequently, the communication needs interpreting, and the factors influencing the communication need to be accounted for.

Chapter 2 develops further discussion on other key concepts, such as environment, that influence the context of care and the impact these can have on communication in an interpersonal setting.

Relationship between communication and interpersonal skills

Well-practised communication techniques alone are ineffectual if the central notion of the interpersonal connection goes unacknowledged. The primary factor, in the nursing context, is the relationship between nurse and patient, co-worker or carer. We are unlikely to communicate without some form of relationship, whether through an information leaflet or poster where there is an intention to relate to persons who may or may not be known, or by physically being close to a person in a bed or chair who is in need of support to prevent suffering, or through a lifesaving intervention or information to prevent further deterioration of a health-related problem. In this light Charlton et al. (2008) differentiate between two different communication styles in the literature they reviewed. These were biomedical and biopsychosocial. The biomedical concentrated on giving specific information on details concerning the patient's condition and are information-focused. The biopsychosocial style is identified as patient-centred communication and this style had a more demonstrable impact on patient outcomes.

Jones (2007) maintains that there is little research in nursing literature that discusses interpersonal skills, particularly in nursing education, whereas there is a rich supply of communication skills research and literatures. This is despite research and policy that have promoted patient-centred communication as effective. There is also a critique that nursing education is often removed from the realities that students experience during their clinical practice, and a lack of literature on CIPS in nursing situations in the clinical environment.

Essential communication skills are deemed to be listening and attending, empathy, information giving, and support in the context of a **therapeutic relationship**. The focus needs to be person-centred rather than nurse- or task-focused and the relationship is a key element. Time spent developing this key relationship is an investment and yet often a precious commodity. Busy wards with high-dependency patients are the norm in many acute care settings, and any time spent in understanding the patient's individual needs is indispensable (McCabe and Timmins, 2006).

Specific areas of nursing specialty require tailored approaches to CIPS, for example in palliative care, in care of the dying, or with children, persons with mental or physical disabilities or patients with learning difficulties. Different settings, such as accident and emergency or intensive care, long-stay wards, clinics and community settings will all require different or particular approaches to CIPS. It is the responsibility of the nurse to identify where these specific needs may be. There is literature and research available in all these areas of practice. A good habit to develop is familiarity with literature searching so that you can find the resources you need to help you with specific settings or care groups. Some of these areas will be covered later in this book. You may be dealing with individuals or groups, for short or long periods of time and in intense emotional situations or circumstances where emotional distance is required. The variety and range of situations are almost infinite.

ASSESSMENT OF PRACTICE

You might want to search the literature for articles on communicating with specific care groups when you are in practice to add to your practice assessment portfolio.

This discussion is therefore implying that there are varying forms of interpersonal proximity and degrees of intensity, purpose and significance that make up the interpersonal aspects of communication in nursing. We are using communication methods from the moment we are born, beginning with the intimacy of the parent–infant interaction, through to the more diffuse connections we have with social networks or in public places such as on the bus each morning travelling to work. Developing our CIPS effectively in different circumstances and with different people has helped us to hone our skills. There is a difference between the social situation and the professional; in the latter there is more at stake if we are ineffective with these skills.

Caring and nursing

Caring is nursing, and nursing is caring.

(Leininger, 1984)

The concept of caring in nursing was a subject of intense interest in the latter decades of the twentieth century (Clarke and Wheeler, 1992; Kyle, 1995). From a perspective that takes into account cultural similarities and differences across individuals and populations, Leininger (1981, 1994) argued that caring in nursing is about the provision of comfort, concern and support, the development of trust and the alleviation of stress. Clearly, whether practised across or within cultures, caring can only be demonstrated when people interact with each other – hence its connection to CIPS.

Interest in conceptualising and defining the concept of caring has developed since the late 1980s. Morse et al. (1991) undertook a detailed analysis of the concept and identified five major areas. They saw caring as:

- a human trait;
- a moral imperative;
- an affect;
- an interpersonal interaction;
- a therapeutic intervention.

Radsma (1994), like Leininger (1984) and Brykczynska (1997), considers caring to be an integral component of nursing, although Radsma claims that nurses have a dilemma in explaining and justifying the significance, meaning and function of nursing care because they believe it to be so integral to everything that they do. Benner and Wrubel (1988), Clarke and Wheeler (1992), Lea et al. (1998) and Kitson (2003) are all examples of empirical studies identifying the components of caring actions in nursing and have helped to articulate what the elements of caring are, in order to bring them into the real world and away from abstract conceptualisation.

Benner et al. (1996) described caring practice in several domains:

- the helping role;
- teaching-coaching functions;
- diagnostic and patient-monitoring functions;
- effective management of rapidly changing situations;
- administering and monitoring therapeutic interventions and regimens.

These are very different from those described by Watson's (1988) transpersonal theory. This theory is organised around concepts such as transpersonalism, phenomenology, the self and the caring occasion, with ten curative factors that guide nursing care. Watson's theory is intended to encompass the whole of nursing; however, it places most emphasis on the experiential, interpersonal processes between the caregiver and recipient. It focuses on caring as a therapeutic relationship and attempts to reduce the components of caring to describable parts, so that these parts can be understood and learned. As such, the theory could be criticised for being reductionist. Watson believes that nursing is *a human-to-human relationship in which the person of nurse affects and is affected by the person of the other* (1988, p58). This might usefully be regarded as 'relational caring' (Hartrick, 1997). Hartrick suggests that more emphasis should be placed on relationship development than on skills development.

The emphasis is now turning to the phenomenon of caring in practice (Spichiger et al., 2005) and to exploring the notion of commitment and the difference between technical care that is embedded in practice and care that attempts to attune itself to actions engaged with others using experience, perceptiveness and an understanding of the responses of others.

Bach (2004) researched the relationship between psychology and caring, and found that there were distinct characteristics that patients found nurses provided in what they described as 'psychological care' – characteristics that were similar to the therapeutic activities of formal psychological care. The nurse–patient relationship was crucial to carrying out this care and a model was devised to capture those activities that are often referred to as 'unseen' or 'invisible' care. The essential themes of unseen care are represented as if refracted from a prism that is usually transparent, and is a parallelogram (representing both pairs of opposite sides as parallel in the nurse–patient/client relationship; see Figure 1.1).

Figure 1.1: Psychological care.

ACTIVITY 1.4   **PRACTICAL**

Can you remember an encounter with someone you know and who you were caring for? Describe the components of that encounter from both your and the other person's perspective. Use the model in Figure 1.1 to guide you. Are they similar?

Compare this with an encounter with someone you do not know. What differences did you find between the two encounters?

As this activity is based on your own reflection, there is no outline answer at the end of the chapter.

The notion that caring is invisible, but 'felt' or experienced by both parties in the relationship, is not new. Watson's (1988) transpersonal theory also features this phenomenon; however, Bach (2004) has illuminated the elements that nurses described in the caring relationship, and that were corroborated by patients from a variety of settings, so that the elements of the interaction have definition. This moves the elements of the interaction from the abstract to the tangible, which means they are more easily understood and integrated into practice. By describing the elements in a more distinct, non-ambiguous and noticeable manner, the interaction can be more effective, which is also the aim of improving CIPS in nursing and caring contexts.

A systematic framework for communication and interpersonal skills

The framework we explore in this section is a universal, cyclical approach that can be used in many different situations and settings. It is a framework you may wish to use in other contexts in which you find yourself during your years as a student, whether this is in acute care or a community setting or clinic, and with any patient/client group (see Figure 1.1). In this chapter we will use it as an overarching guide to communication and interpersonal encounters in nursing. Figure 1.2 gives an outline of the five stages.

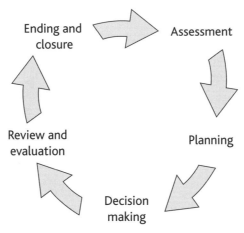

Figure 1.2: Being systematic.

Assessment

This is the first stage of the process and involves gathering relevant information, developing an overview of the general situation and thinking about what needs to be done. It is also the preparatory stage for deciding whether to intervene in a situation, an intermediate stage to review or evaluate what has happened so far, or an end-of-care encounter to determine to what extent the intended outcomes of a situation have been met. It is important to note that, while an assessment is often a preliminary activity and will be written down and recorded, it is not just a bureaucratic exercise and is part of a process that is often cyclical.

ACTIVITY 1.5   PRACTICAL

In your next placement, look for the assessment tools that are used in the department. What do you think is important about these tools in relation to CIPS. Are they very long, too detailed or about right? Are they active documents –

---

referred to by both the staff on the unit and the patients, and are they specific to the unit or generic health assessments? Ask the qualified staff for their views on the assessments and then ask a patient, if this is possible. Compare the two viewpoints.

As this activity is based on your own practice, there is no outline answer at the end of the chapter.

Key issues in assessment

From a CIPS perspective, assessment begins with a consideration of a person's 'social location'. Key aspects to consider are:

- race and likelihood of being exposed to racism;
- ethnicity – particular cultural or religious needs;
- gender – whether sexism is relevant to the situation;
- language – whether an interpreter is needed;
- disability – whether there is a physical or mental impairment;
- age – whether there are generational issues to respect and consider or any developmental needs.

Are there legislative and policy requirements to acknowledge? For example, what are you empowered to do by legislation, what are the contractual duties you are expected to perform, and what limitations are there that restrict you in responding to the situation? You may want to discuss this with your mentor.

The next step is to gather information using appropriate methods of communication. We will be looking at the exact skills later in this book. However, you will need to think about your non-verbal as well as verbal skills and consider the interpersonal dynamics of power and authority between the nurse and the patient. For example, are you paying due deference to the patient by seeking permissions or consents, is there a balance of contribution to the communication, is the patient being excluded from contributing or is the patient being spoken for? Who will be making the ultimate decisions about the nursing interventions and are there reasons why the intervention may not be negotiated between the professionals and the patient?

A common mistake is to gather as much information as possible, but this is problematic. It could be an intrusion into a person's privacy and has trust been established? Gathering more information than necessary could be a waste of valuable time. Being flooded with more information than necessary could confound the picture and reduce clarity for planning.

A central feature is confidentiality. Environments in many settings are not conducive to maintaining this aspect; however, efforts to maintain privacy should be made if at all possible. Also, there are some circumstances where information belongs to the organisation rather than the individual, for example in situations of suspected abuse.

Always seek guidance in these situations from a qualified person. The aim should be to state clearly to patients how the information they provide is likely to be recorded and used.

Always attempt to separate fact from opinion. It is probable that both will be gleaned in any assessment to get a whole picture. However, opinion may be wrong and should be verified as a fact before any intervention is taken. In emotional situations, fears, worries, anxieties and even exhilaration can distort facts and these circumstances need careful management to gain an exact assessment of a situation.

Avoid jargon and vague terms that can confuse the patient. Establish their level of understanding of any unusual terms. Be clear to yourself and the patient about how the information you are gathering will feed into any plan of action. Link the information you are gathering into potential and realistic timescales, as this will give the patient a sense of points in time and priority.

Well-conducted assessments using the full range of CIPS skills are complex and require patience, skill, clear thinking and vision. At the end of the assessment process sufficient information is gathered to form a clear picture of the problem(s) requiring intervention(s). It is helpful to set out aims or objectives of what is to be achieved at this stage. This is the planning stage.

Planning

This stage in nursing is usually related to setting out the physical actions that need to take place to improve a situation, such as arranging tests, preparation for procedures, administering treatments, and giving information or education on conditions and management of situations. From a CIPS perspective, planning is focused on less tangible factors and is more concerned with establishing the direction and meaning that a plan of action will have for a person; meeting the needs and effects of any unmet needs; establishing the impact a plan will have on a person's place in life, developmentally or socially; identifying the motivators and reasons for acting out a plan; establishing a 'psychological contract' or agreement to continue with the plan; and the involvement or sign-up of other professionals, co-workers or carers in the plan. This is a stage of explanation, exploration, negotiation and agreement.

CASE STUDY

Sheila was a woman in her fifties who had developed severe congestive cardiac failure. Her husband had died a year earlier from bowel cancer and her three children, although all adults and supportive of her, had their own families and children that consumed much of their time. Sheila became very depressed and was reluctant to take her medication. She felt she had lost all sense of purpose and her life had lost its direction and meaning.

She was desperate to have a purposeful role back in her life, as she perceived that she was no longer a mother or wife, which had been pivotal roles for her. She could not see that she could become involved in her grandparenting role and that, although her condition was serious, the medication could help her to fulfil her life and maximise her contribution to her children's lives. The plan would also be to help her manage her medications, so that they would become part of her life and not take over, thus shifting the focus from dependence to independence.

Her family were approached, with her permission, to participate in the plan to help her re-evaluate her life and find suitable activities and occasions for her to help with the grandchildren. Her progress could be monitored by her GP or practice nurse.

A basic component of planning is to understand the roles and responsibilities of others collaborating in the plan as well as what will be expected of the patient. There will be different values and priorities to consider from different professional groups. Professional hierarchies can sometimes become obstructive where rivalry and power bids detract from the essential aim of the planning process. Partnership should therefore be the aim, not hierarchies.

Decision making

The logical conclusion of any assessment and planning is to make a decision about how to proceed, because it is unrealistic for anyone to carry out a plan by simply following instructions. This stage is therefore an analysis of how effective the plan will be and the success of subsequent interventions. This will involve weighing up the pros and cons of the facts, and their value or priority in any situation, as well as the worth given to the actions in the plan and subsequent interventions. Decision making in the context of CIPS is to think about the significance and consequence of decisions for patients as well as estimate the perceived risks and levels of uncertainty. This can impact on adherence to treatment and the success of interventions.

The decision-making process is about evaluating options to decide the best course of action. First, all the options have to be described. The questions to ask are as follows.

- What obstacles are there in relation to each option?
- What risks are involved?
- How can these be removed or minimised?
- Which decisions are feasible?
- Which of these offer a realistic chance of success?
- How attractive are the available options?
- Does one simple decision need to be made or can a combination of decisions be made?
- What timeframe are we working to?
- What might we need to do to keep options open for the future?
- How well does the decision fit in with existing strategies?

Not all of these questions need to be answered; however, they can usefully clarify any problems ahead and how they can be addressed. Decision making is weighing up what can and cannot be achieved, deciding on the best plan of action and how to achieve success in an outcome. It is a stage that is often overlooked.

Review and evaluation

Review is a process that takes place during any intervention and involves standing back and judging the effectiveness of what has been planned. It is a process of monitoring and checking. Evaluation, however, is identifying the strengths and weaknesses of the assessment and intervention stages at an end point.

There are three questions to ask in a review of any situation.

1. What are you trying to achieve?
2. How are you going to achieve it?
3. How will you know when you have achieved it?

To answer these questions you have to consider if the original objectives were appropriate and if there remain any obstacles to achieving the desired outcome. There may have been subtle and gradual changes in the situation, so the plan may need to be reviewed in this light.

Evaluation seeks to measure how effective any intervention has been against the original aims or objectives. A judgement can also be made on the efficiency of the plan and the use of people's time and resources. Did the nurse spend too long talking to Mr Smith about his post-operative recovery period, in order to reduce his anxieties? Alternatively, did the nurse not spend enough time with the parents of a child who needed emergency interventions for an acute asthma attack, in order to explain what was happening and the potential outcome? In particular, in CIPS, the extent of human resources, such as emotions and personal value constructs, needs to be considered. Evaluation in the nursing context takes account of moral and professional requirements as well as principles of good practice. We are constantly aiming to improve our performance to identify mistakes, so that they can be avoided in future, and so that we can enhance professional credibility, provide opportunities for learning for ourselves and others, and maintain our professional and personal development.

Ending and closure

The termination of our involvement with a particular person or patients is an important factor in CIPS. It is more than saying goodbye or tying up loose ends. Effective endings can reduce the likelihood of further problems arising if, for example, anticipatory information is given about likely future problems, resources for self-management, advice and education.

Endings can be inhibited by dependency on healthcare staff, resistance to change, satisfaction with working with particular groups, thus creating reluctance to move on, or pressure from others to stay with patients because that presence is deemed to prevent problems recurring. Certain situations can trigger emotional responses and echoes of previous ones and, if it was a pleasurable time, it may be difficult to end such an association. Failing to review objectives can result in staying too long with a problem situation and, finally, poor time management and a disorganised approach to workload can work against effective planning to find the appropriate time and words to end an association.

ACTIVITY 1.6   REFLECTIVE

Think of a time when you felt very comfortable with a patient or family of a patient whom you had helped through a long recovery process. You had gained a sense of achievement from helping and had grown fond of the patient – a not unreasonable feeling. How did you end that association when the time came for them to be discharged? Were you able to let go and take account of your personal feelings and not let them affect the situation?

As this activity is based on your own reflection, there is no outline answer at the end of the chapter.

CHAPTER SUMMARY

This is the first chapter in this book on communication and interpersonal skills (CIPS). The chapter has set the scene for the nursing context of CIPS. It has examined the issues facing nursing today in achieving effective and safe CIPS. The two concepts of 'communication' and 'interpersonal skills' have been explored and differentiated. The caring domain of nursing as a context for improving CIPS has been examined. Finally, a systematic framework for CIPS in nursing has been described to demonstrate how a methodical approach, which includes analysing factors influencing the process of CIPS, can improve nursing care decisions and outcomes.

Activities: brief outline answers

As the results of all the activities in this chapter are based on your own observations and decision-making abilities, there are no outline answers for this chapter.

KNOWLEDGE REVIEW

Having completed the chapter, how would you now rate your knowledge of the following topics?

	Good	Adequate	Poor
1. The two main different types of communication.			
2. The difference between 'communication' and 'interpersonal skills' and why they need to overlap in nursing.			
3. What caring in nursing means and the essential elements.			
4. The main features of a systematic approach to CIPS.			

Where you're not confident in your knowledge of a topic, what will you do next?

Further reading

Chambers, C and Ryder, E (2009) *Compassion and Caring in Nursing*. Oxford: Radcliffe Publishing.

Useful websites

www.culturediversity.org/basic.htm This site will introduce you to Leininger's theory of transcultural nursing. This is a humanistic and scientific area of formal study and practice in nursing, which is focused on differences and similarities among cultures with respect to human care, health and illness, based on people's cultural values, beliefs and practices. The intention is to promote the use of this knowledge to provide cultural specific or culturally congruent nursing care to people.

www.nursing.ucdenver.edu/faculty/caring.htm This site will introduce you to the theory of caring science and the foundations of Watson's transpersonal theory. The theory was developed to bring meaning and focus to nursing and make explicit nursing's values, knowledge and practices of human caring that are geared towards subjective inner healing processes. It is based on the notion of cherishing.

Both these websites demonstrate the author's work in these two major nursing theories. You will revisit these theories in later chapters.

2. Key concepts

CHAPTER AIMS

After reading this chapter, you will be able to:

- understand the crucial need for effective and sophisticated interpersonal communication in modern healthcare organisations;

- define and explain good communication and interpersonal skills (CIPS);

- understand the frameworks underpinning good interpersonal communication;

- explain why good interpersonal communication makes a significant difference to nursing practice;

- differentiate between CIPS in nursing and in counselling and psychotherapy;

- outline the evidence base for CIPS in nursing;

- describe the nursing, and related, theories underpinning interpersonal communication in nursing;

- describe the organisational basis for healthy interpersonal relating in nursing.

Introduction

Because we all believe we are good at communicating, we think there is no need to think about how we do it. Yet, regrettably, there is ample literature to suggest that we do not communicate as well as we might in healthcare settings. In this chapter, we will be exploring those ideas and trying to come to terms with the notion that we can rise to the challenge of improving CIPS interactions in our different spheres of practice.

The NMC *Standards of Proficiency* (2004a) stress that nurses should commit themselves to lifelong learning, safely and effectively extend the scope of their professional practice and think in a future-directed and nursing branch-related way. According to the NMC, this commitment should be made within the full range of, often highly different, multidisciplinary team workplaces. These workplaces should promote safety and responsiveness to the needs of the patients and clients within them.

What would a commitment to these standards mean for the healthcare organisations, and the nurses working in them, that were sensitive to the need for the development of increasingly effective and sophisticated interpersonal communication for nurses and midwives? Writers such as Benner et al. (cited in Frost et al., 2000), for example, argue that CIPS are on just as much a continuum from 'novice' to 'expert' as are technical nursing skills. Benner and colleagues argue that highly proficient nurses demonstrate the ability for 'emotional attunement' with their clients. In the context of safe, effective and compassionate organisational work settings, this means that:

> *Attuned nurses have a capacity to read a situation in a patient and to grasp its emotional tone: to know when something is 'off' when it looks 'ok' on the surface, or to sense that it's actually 'ok' despite appearances to the contrary.*
>
> (Frost et al., 2000, p32)

CASE STUDY

The community nurse

A community nurse visits one of her patients to dress her leg ulcer. She does this on a regular basis and usually finds her patient cheerful and engaging. On this particular day, however, she notices that her patient, although apparently pleasant and cheerful as usual, seems 'off'. The nurse doesn't receive any obvious signs to tell her that something is wrong with her patient, but has a 'gut feeling' that something is not right. She spends more time than usual with her patient and, over a cup of tea, sensitively and gently questions her about what might be wrong. The patient discloses that her husband has recently become unwell with suspected heart problems. This has been worrying her since the nurse's last visit.

To help improve our CIPS, theorists have explored the manner in which we communicate and relate to one another to provide us with explanations for why and how we carry out what could be considered a fundamental human behaviour. In this chapter, we will consider some of these theories and how they apply to healthcare settings. We will also examine why evidence and research underpinning our practice needs to be determined in this area in line with current thinking on the strength of this evidence.

There are questions to ask about how well we consider our abilities to communicate and, in this chapter, we will ask these questions. Because there are so many different factors that can affect our ability to communicate, we will be concentrating here on what we believe to be two very important aspects: how we can better understand relating to one another in a healthy manner and how we can understand each other's emotional needs and perceptions. This latter aspect involves considering the caring element of communication and the notion of suffering; each firmly situated in healthcare. We move on to discuss the psychological basis for healthy relationships by exploring the theory of mind, empathy and the notion of valuing diversity.

The final section of the chapter concentrates on the environmental context and discusses the organisational context for CIPS, as well as offering a challenging view on nurses' and midwives' responsibilities to practise quality communication when healthcare environments are subject to change and shifting priorities.

Exploring the definitions

There are many texts written for nurses that seek to explain CIPS. Definitions in the therapeutic communication skills literature generally vary from the apparently highly technical and impersonal to the more human. Consider the following examples and make a decision about the one or ones that appeal to you most, and the reasons for its/their appeal:

> *Communication is about the reciprocal process in which messages are sent and received between two or more people.*
>
> (Balzer-Riley, 2004)

> *Interpersonal communication involves a series of messages or information which people send out to, and receive from, each other through the use of the senses, such as seeing, touching and hearing one another.*
>
> (Petrie, 1997)

> *Communication is a universal function of humankind, independent of any place, time or context.*
>
> (Ruesch, 1961)

What kinds of factors influenced your choice? Is communication between people, or interpersonal communication, simply and only a functional part of life – undertaken to get things done? Or is communication, in addition to its practical purposes, more about enriching the quality of our lives as individuals and in groups?

> *I don't need to work at developing communication and interpersonal skills. They come naturally.*

This is a commonly expressed view among some students new to nursing. How true is it? Read the following paragraphs on communication frameworks and then ask yourself this question again.

Communication frameworks

Communication is considered a basic tool in healthcare relationships. However, the quality of the communication has a strong relationship to its effectiveness. There are two theoretical frameworks describing how communication takes place: the linear and the circular or transactional. The linear model involves communication from a sender to a receiver via a message (see Table 2.1). The message is relayed by one or more of the five senses (sight, touch, hearing, taste or smell).

A more modern addition to this rather simplistic model is to consider communication as a circular rather than linear process and a process that takes account of a larger social system and context. The model was originally developed by Bateson (1979) and still has relevance today as it takes account of the effects of the context within

Table 2.1: Linear framework of communication.

Sender →	Message →	Receiver
Idea is encoded and expressed.	Verbal and/or non-verbal thoughts and/or feelings.	Idea is decoded, translated into words or symbols and made sense of.
Sender has the responsibility for accuracy of the content and emotional tone.		

which an interaction takes place. Communication is viewed as being continuous, involving mutual giving and receiving. It is an expansion of the linear model and uses a systems approach to understanding communication. In systems models each part has an effect on another part in the system. The sender and receiver each has a set of characteristics that influence the communication. There are shared characteristics for both, which are: culture, knowledge, communication abilities and style, values, internal frame of reference and role. The sender has a set of factors that relate to their needs and goals, and their communication style and abilities influence the communication. The receiver also has goals and needs, but added to this are their previous experiences and any support systems that they may have or will have (see Figure 2.1).

This model emphasises the complexity of communication and the many factors that have to be taken into account. It also indicates that the ability of the communicator has a significant effect and the internal value systems of the individuals involved in communicating with each other play a part. There is also a strong hint in this model that it is not just communicating that enables messages to be transmitted. The interpersonal nature of one person's response to another person counts. The situational context in which the interaction takes place also has an effect.

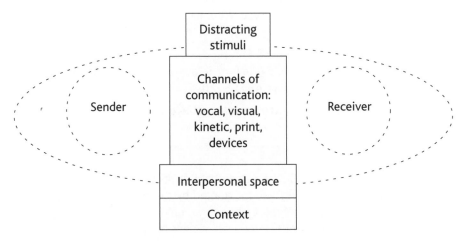

Figure 2.1: Circular transactional framework of communication.

It should become clear from reading the rest of this chapter and the book as a whole that some people are better at communicating than others. If skilled interpersonal communication involves both giving and receiving information, and doing this to the mutual satisfaction and benefit of sender and receiver, then not everyone is 'naturally' very good at:

- figuring out what an individual is feeling from the way they look;
- getting a clear verbal message across so that someone understands it;
- gauging someone else's level of distress on the basis of what they say or how they appear;
- listening respectfully to the experiences and point of view of another person.

Given the above, it should hopefully be clear that the ability to be interpersonally skilled communicators cannot be taken for granted by student nurses or midwives. We wish to explode the myth that these skills come naturally to human beings and require no effort to constantly hone, improve and develop them.

ACTIVITY 2.3   **PRACTICAL**

Conduct an informal survey among either your student peers or your colleagues on the ward or placement. Ask either group what makes for good communication between staff and between staff and clients. Keep a brief written record of this exercise and share it in class.

As this activity is based on your own observations, there is no outline answer at the end of the chapter.

Do communication and interpersonal skills make a difference?

From a number of sources – including ordinary human experience, CIPS research (Hargie and Dickson, 2004) and psychotherapy research (Gilbert and Leahy, 2007) – there is every reason to accept that the skilful practice of CIPS makes a positive, healing difference to clients and patients. Specifically, this includes patients/clients:

- feeling listened to;
- feeling that their concerns are being validated and not trivialised;
- feeling supported;
- feeling understood.

CASE STUDY

The community psychiatric nurse

A community psychiatric nurse pays a regular visit to one of his clients who is housebound because of mobility problems. Because his client has very little contact with the outside world, or with people other than his community psychiatric nurse, he values his visits as they give him a chance to talk about how he has been feeling and the difficulties he has been experiencing since the last visit. The community psychiatric nurse sees the main purpose of his visits as simply to listen to his client, and to demonstrate empathy, and that he has fully understood and takes his client's concerns seriously.

Skills in nursing and skills in counselling and psychotherapy

A distinction should be made at this point between good CIPS within nursing practice and their use in the two other disciplines of counselling and psychotherapy.

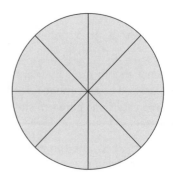

| In counselling and psychotherapy, the therapeutic relationship radiates throughout the interactions between counsellor/therapist and client. | In nursing care, communication is one element of several that make up holistic nursing practice. |

Figure 2.2: Difference between therapeutic relationships in counselling and psychotherapy and in nursing care.

There are some similarities, but equally there are many differences (see Figure 2.2). All three disciplines aim to make helpful and effective use of CIPS. However, the therapeutic relationship in counselling and psychotherapy is viewed as central and pivotal, rather than being just one element of the many role aspects that go to make up the job of nursing. In addition, issues emerging within the therapeutic relationship between client and psychotherapist or counsellor are worked on in considerably greater depth and sophistication, and treated with much greater significance than they would be in a nurse–client/patient relationship (see, for example, Gilbert and Leahy, 2007).

Evidence-based communication and interpersonal skills

The NMC *Standards of Proficiency* (2004a) argue that nursing practice, integrated with theory, needs to be evidence-based, and thus safe. There are good reasons why the safe and effective practice of CIPS in nursing should aim to be evidence-based (the specific focus of Chapter 3). From a broad definition of evidence-based nursing, practices are considered safe and effective either because of a developing body of research-based scientific (sometimes called 'empirical') knowledge to support them, or because of theoretical consensus.

'Theoretical consensus' means large-scale agreement, built up over a long time, by communities of nursing practitioners and academics, and scholars from outside the discipline whose work has been seen to have relevance for nursing.

Together, researchers and theorists have contributed to the *systematic* consideration about, reflection on, and refinement of nursing CIPS practice. This contrasts strongly with the notion of simply relating to, and communicating with, patients and clients in particular styles because 'it's always been done that way' or because it's 'quick and easy'. This also points to CIPS in nursing with people having healthcare needs as being distinct from everyday communication between people in general.

The box that follows will introduce you to key fundamental issues around evidence-based healthcare practice, and the section and activities that follow this box will help you begin to engage with some systematically developed theoretical and scientific concerns.

THEORY SUMMARY

Evidence-based healthcare

Healthcare practice should be based on the combination of three factors (Muir Gray, 1997; Trinder and Reynolds, 2000). These are:

- the best available evidence;
- the values of society;
- the resources available.

The practice of evidence-based healthcare is conducted on the basis of an established hierarchy of strength of evidence, described below, where 1 is assumed to be the source of evidence that healthcare practitioners can place the most confidence in (Muir Gray, 1997):

1. Strong evidence from at least one systematic review of multiple and well-designed randomised control trials.
2. Strong evidence from at least one properly designed randomised control trial of an appropriate size.
3. Evidence from well-designed research trials that do not contain randomisation, for example single-group, pre-post, cohort, time series or matched case-control studies.
4. Evidence from well-designed non-experimental studies from more than one centre or research group.
5. Opinions of respected authorities, based on clinical evidence, descriptive studies, reports or expert committees.

ACTIVITY 2.4   REFLECTIVE

With a fellow group of students, consider what the range of challenges might be with regard to implementing evidence-based CIPS in either adult or mental health nursing work settings.

You will find possible answers to this activity at the end of the chapter.

Underpinning nursing, and related, theories

A question may be raised by some of you at this stage about why safe, effective, evidence-based CIPS *should* have a theoretical base to justify their practice. Earlier in this chapter, you hopefully saw the problems with the viewpoint that 'communication skills are simply common sense. Everybody has them, so they don't need to be learnt'.

Accepting that these skills need to be worked on over the lifespan of a nursing career, within organisations that deserve the title of truly caring, several nurse scholar-practitioners and scholars from disciplines other than nursing have, over the years, provided a theoretical foundation that is arguably indispensable.

There are many strands to this foundation and we will go on to help you explore two that we think are most relevant. These are **suffering** and *four aspects of **healthy relating***. Sometimes, such strands have developed from systematic reviews of nursing and related literature, which look for key arguments or how concepts have been used and developed in nursing over the years. Equally, sometimes strands are identified from quantitative or qualitative scientific research. Quantitative research refers to conducting experiments to arrive at helpful outcomes, while qualitative research involves searching for meanings and experiences by talking with, and listening to, patients or nursing staff individually or in groups, or by observing them interacting together.

What all the strands have in common is a concern for the ongoing, ethically important, development of 'moral' practice (Armstrong, 2006; Clay and Povey, 1983; Wurzbach, 1999). Quite simply, **moral practice** amounts to believing that 'good' and 'right' practice is more to be desired than practice that is 'bad' and 'wrong'.

Suffering

Interpersonal sensitivity, used in the service of helping others within a trusting relationship, must be linked to a sensitivity to the suffering of others. From a review of the literature, undertaken to help nurses gain a better conceptual understanding of this area, Rodgers and Cowles (1997) argued that suffering is a complex concept that cannot be readily observed or measured. According to these authors, its individual and subjective nature means that it is uniquely experienced by each individual.

However, there are clear similarities between people who are suffering. First, they show high levels of distress in relation to their physical or mental anguish. Second, suffering individuals place negative meanings in the situations in which they find themselves. These negative meanings may be influenced by the need to guard against the socially stigmatising effects of living with visible or invisible chronic physical conditions or mental health difficulties. Two key words are particularly important to the experience of suffering, as described above. These are **loss** and **control**:

> *According to the authors of the literature examined, the meaning that characterises suffering is quite profound, involving a tremendous sense of the loss of the person's integrity, autonomy, or control over his or her situation or life . . . In*

suffering, individuals can be thought of as being in the process of losing their very 'humanity', and all the things that are considered to be related to humanness and dignity.

(Rodgers and Cowles, 1997, p1050)

ACTIVITY 2.5   REFLECTIVE

Based on your observation of a suffering patient/client and your own response to their suffering:

- What could be inferred about how the individual experienced their suffering?
- What communication/interpersonal interventions were helpful/would be helpful/were needed?

As this activity is based on your own observations, there is no outline answer at the end of the chapter.

Healthy relating

From the chapter so far, we can make the following summary statements: good CIPS in nursing are respectful, non-exploitative, non-judgemental and not tainted by everyday casualness. They must be based on the careful development of sensitive helping-trusting relationships with individuals who are suffering because of their perceived loss, and loss of control, of functions, abilities and other attributes that make them human and give them dignity.

However, the above picture of the basis in nursing theory for good, effective and safe CIPS can be broadened with reference to the NMC *Standards of Proficiency* (2004a). The health promotion and education roles of nurses and midwives include a focus that goes beyond a narrow disease orientation to address 'healthy relating'. Healthy relating, in turn, has a developmental basis, a moral basis, a psychological basis and an organisational basis. We will go on to examine each of these now.

The developmental basis for healthy relating

According to Bowlby (1988), relationships between adults mirror the kinds of 'attachment' relationships that can occur between infants and their primary caregivers. In Bowlby's terms, healthy relational living can be described as a series of excursions from a secure base. In **unhealthy relating**, individuals avoid such excursions for fear of abandonment or the removal of their secure base.

There are clear implications emerging from such 'healthy' and 'unhealthy' attachment styles for interpersonal communication between nurses and midwives and their patients or clients. Arguably the most important of these is that patients may need to be helped to feel reasonably secure in their relationship with nurses. This is achieved through nurses and midwives offering their patients and clients time, within which they listen non-judgementally to those they care for. From the perspective of secure relationships, more healthily attached individuals, who feel listened to, understood and supported, will be more able to take risks towards independent living and increased health.

ACTIVITY 2.6   REFLECTIVE

- With your peers, think of children you knew when you were very young. Can you distinguish between those who were timid and shy and those who were very confident 'natural leaders'? How might their respective home and parental environments have contributed to their shyness and confidence?

- Think of people you know currently. Can you distinguish between 'non-risk-takers' and 'risk-takers'? Is there anything about the early lives of each group that may have contributed to their current respective styles around risk?

Apply the two scenario questions above to clients/patients that you know.

What kinds of relationships with healthcare staff might help clients or patients feel enabled to take risks towards independent living and increased health?

As this activity is based on your own observations and discussions, there is no outline answer at the end of the chapter.

The moral basis for healthy relating

The provision of time to be listened to, by nurses and midwives, may be something of a novelty for some patients. One reason for this is that they have gone through their lives being treated as objects in various ways. This could include being treated as a *precious object* who must not be damaged in any way, or an *unwanted object* whose presence is a constant nuisance, or a *useless object* who can do nothing right.

The work of the philosopher Martin Buber (1958) is helpful in understanding the ethical basis for healthy relationships. In simplified form, Buber's argument is that we all have a choice to relate to each other either as objects (what he terms 'I–It') or as full human beings ('I–Thou'). Full human relating amounts to the ethical practice of respectful attention to, and respect for, the inner world, feelings, beliefs and viewpoints of the other person.

ACTIVITY 2.7   REFLECTIVE

What makes you feel as if you are being treated as a person, and that your individual needs are being recognised and regarded as valued? Write down your ideas and think about whether or not these are the same as your friends' or family's.

As this activity is based on your own reflection, there is no outline answer at the end of the chapter.

Using Buber's terminology, the experience of being treated as an 'I' rather than an 'it' is more likely to lead to individuals feeling self-confident and independent and trusting their own worth, judgement and feelings. This in turn may well help them to begin to develop more healthy relationships, both with themselves, in terms of having greater **self-esteem**, and with others.

THEORY SUMMARY

Self-esteem

Self-esteem reflects the emotions that result from individuals' appraisal of their overall effectiveness in the conduct of their lives (Hewitt, 1998). Self-esteem is thus clearly subjective and develops from a person's perceptions of themselves and their achievements. This is particularly so in interpersonal relationships and relates to the value and significance we place on our views of ourselves – or our self-concept.

To complicate matters, a person may have many objective achievements and still have a low self-esteem. Conversely, a person with few achievements who believes they have conducted themselves as well as they could can have a high self-esteem.

In healthcare there is often a lowering of self-esteem because the person is unable to function as they would normally. They may previously have had a satisfactory level of self-esteem or an ability to aspire to achieve higher levels. Yet levels of self-esteem can be maintained through ill-health if patients are given the appropriate levels of support. This works in two ways. Either a person's health creates such a threat to their self-identity that they become emotionally immobilised. Or they will be sufficiently challenged by the illness or change in health that they develop new coping skills that result in an increase in self-esteem. The nurse's role is to provide support and confirmation of the person's efforts to help protect their self-esteem.

ACTIVITY 2.8   REFLECTIVE

With a group of fellow students or friends, think about the following questions and ask your group what they think and discuss their responses. In this way you not only reflect on your own views on self-esteem, but begin to hear about other people's perceptions of self-esteem and its meaning to them.

- In general, what kind of actions do you think enhance self-esteem?
- What are some things (actions or words or both) that people do that diminish self-esteem?
- What specific things in healthcare settings do you think you can do to enhance self-esteem for patients and colleagues?
- What did you learn about yourself from this exercise?

As this activity is based on your own observations, there is no outline answer at the end of the chapter.

The psychological basis for healthy relating

Some individuals who have experienced a lifetime of being mistreated, and who therefore regard themselves in Buber's terms as an 'it', have from a very young age had their inner world of meanings and feelings constantly disregarded by those who have been in the closest contact with them. Those in closest contact with young children are normally their parents and, a little later, their teachers and peers at school. The influence of these close contacts can have a considerable effect on a person's psychological well-being and sense of self-esteem and self-worth. These ideas and interpretations of the meanings of experiences with others form the basis of an individual's own theory of concepts and imaginations – reasons why things happen the way they do around them or to them. This is known as the '**theory of mind**' and plays a large part in influencing the psychological basis for healthy relating to others.

THEORY SUMMARY

Theory of mind

In a dynamic interactive way, human beings make constant judgements about each other. The 'theory of mind' concept refers to how all of us make inferences and guesses about what we think are the causes of each other's behaviours, and what is going through each other's minds (Baron-Cohen, 2003; Goleman, 2006).

The human ability to have a theory of mind seems to be important to us in order to 'read' situations well enough to get by relatively smoothly and helpfully with one another on a day-to-day basis. However, theory of mind is a specific skill and some people have major difficulties in being able to guess what is going on in other people's minds. Sometimes, as in the case of how young children are treated by their parents and teachers, it is sadly the case that what's going on in the minds of the former is of little importance to the latter.

The work of Baron-Cohen (2003), although in large part dealing with Asperger's syndrome, has wider implications for the psychological basis of healthy relating

(Goleman, 2006). As with the ability to be empathic, described below, people in general differ in their abilities to judge accurately the internal world of another. This has clear implications for the ongoing development of skilled interpersonal communication in nursing . Nursing students should not assume that they are highly skilled in this area, and may have to work at developing this ability (Goleman, 2006).

Empathy

In addition to understanding the complexity of an individual's personal theory of mind and its impact on CIPS, being empathic requires the ability to not just think about the mind of the other but to identify emotionally with his or her feelings (Greenberg, 2007). Empathy can be described as the ability to be intuitively aware of what another person is feeling as well as thinking.

We believe empathy is the ability of one person to perceive and understand another person's emotions. But this is not easy to do, as emotions can be hidden in an internal world or displayed with behaviours that can contradict how a person actually feels. Such are the complexities of human beings. In a primitive survival setting you would not have wanted your opponent to know what you were feeling, so we have learnt as a species to disguise how we really feel, and this often occurs when we are most distressed.

We have to learn, therefore, how to communicate our understanding of another's feelings through verbal and non-verbal expressions and then (here comes the tricky bit) interpret those signals accurately. In healthcare, this complex interaction takes place in settings that are often far from ideal – for example, on busy wards, being overheard by others, during painful experiences or on hearing bad news.

In these situations, nurses and midwives have to draw upon their professional inner emotional strengths and try to feel the emotions their patient/client feels, while at the same time maintaining a separate identity. It is important to recognise which feelings belong to the patient/client and which to the nurse. This is a difficult skill to learn and Chapter 3 will provide more guidance on how to develop this ability.

Other theoretical concepts to consider when judging and engaging with patients in relation to empathy are *trust* and *respect*. Trust is based upon our previous experiences and enables individuals to cope with the world and resolve frustrations about those things that may be unfamiliar or unknown. Respect, together with honesty, consistency, faith and hope, is an element of a trusting relationship. Once these elements are established, a sharing of emotions and thoughts can take place.

Empathic attunement

Complementing Benner's views on 'emotional attunement' (discussed in the introduction to this chapter) is Greenberg's concept of 'empathic attunement', derived from scientific research. Empathic attunement suggests that nurses and midwives who convey genuine interest, acceptance and caring are more likely to achieve a secure emotional bond with their patients. In this regard, non-verbal facial communication is extremely important. Essentially, patients and clients learn how acceptable they are from the facial expressions of healthcare staff (Greenberg, 2007).

CASE STUDY

The in-patient adult nurse

While sitting by the bedside of one of her patients, the nurse hears a story from the patient's past which makes her feel disturbed and somewhat disgusted. The patient has disclosed that she was sexually abused by her father over several years, when she was very young. Mindful of the importance of facial expression in empathic communication, the nurse makes an effort to match her supportive and sensitive response to the patient's disclosure with a facial expression that signifies care and concern rather than shock and disgust.

Chapter 3 discusses this concept in more detail and examines the evidence underpinning the concept.

Valuing diversity

Practice in developing increasingly honed skills around empathy and theory of mind provides opportunities for nurses to appreciate the fact that other people do not feel and think in the same way as them. It should be apparent that differences in feeling and thinking between people may be based on age, gender, culture, sexual orientation, ethnic origin and, as stated above, upbringing. Chapter 8 explores this area in more detail.

The organisational basis for healthy relating

The above section has hopefully illustrated the importance of nurses and midwives working towards secure rather than insecure attachment styles in their patients and clients, and supporting them in a health-promoting way to believe more in themselves, and in their emotions and judgements. However, the above bases for healthy relationships depend in turn upon healthy and health-promoting work settings. These provide the organisational basis for good CIPS, a discussion of which will bring this chapter to a close.

The NMC *Standards of Proficiency* (2004a) require nurses to be able to engage in problem solving, critical thinking and reflection around safe and effective CIPS within the complex and varied care environments that characterise health provision in the twenty-first century. These behaviours should be carried out in the context of multidisciplinary practice, and be fair, professionally and ethically appropriate, and responsive to the needs of diverse patient/client populations.

Environments shape experience

Sadly, the nature and influence of healthcare organisations is a much neglected area in nursing and health CIPS books. This is surprising, given the strong message emerging from the social psychological literature that organisational environments shape experience (Meyerson, 2002), at both conscious and unconscious levels (Morgan, 1997).

THEORY SUMMARY

External and internal environments

By environment, we mean all the cultural, developmental, physical and psychological features that are external to a person and that can have an influence on their perception, reaction and involvement in healthcare. These are the features that we bring as professionals to the healthcare setting, either as individuals or collectively as part of an organisation.

In addition, we need to consider the effect of the internal environmental state of the patient/client, which is derived from their physiological, spiritual, psychological and developmental characteristics. These internal states will have been influenced by beliefs from family, friends, the media, and any previous experiences they have had of healthcare settings.

Two views of healthcare organisations

Common sense might tell us that the healthcare organisations within which we do our placements are simply the settings where people work together to carry out the delivery of high-quality nursing care. This is sometimes referred to as a 'realist' view of organisations. From this perspective, the work of the people in the organisation is regarded as separate from the organisation itself or from what people think about the organisation.

However, an entirely different picture of healthcare organisations is possible, sometimes referred to as the 'social constructionist' view of organisations. From a social constructionist perspective, the process of thinking and acting together within specific organisational circumstances contributes over time to a social and cultural agreement about 'the way things are done here'.

This view of organisations shifts the focus away from simple 'bricks and mortar' assumptions of what organisations are about. From a realist perspective, organisations are simply physical structures within which employees work. From a social constructionist perspective, organisations are social-psychological structures that individuals create together in their day-to-day interactions.

An unfortunate fact is the reported experience of many clients and patients, often confirmed by staff, of some work settings within which 'the way things are done' is clearly to the disadvantage of the communication and interpersonal needs of patients and clients, in the following ways.

CASE STUDY

The nurse on a ward caring for elderly clients with limited mobility

A young student nurse is on a placement in a nursing home that cares for, often immobile, elderly clients. She notices that the qualified nurses and assistant nurses often don't speak to their clients as they give them bed baths and feed them. This seems to be part of the 'culture' of the home.

Task- versus person-orientation

In clear violation of the ethic of healthy relating, in the senses discussed above, sometimes patients are treated as objects rather than people. This is because the work culture is task- rather than person-oriented, in spite of such things as glossy, locally produced mission statements to the contrary. According to the research and theorising of Menzies Lyth (1988), nursing task-orientation functions as a *social system to defend against anxiety*. From this perspective, it is arguably less demanding to treat patients or clients as 'bodies' to be washed, fed, dressed, etc. rather than as people to be listened to, or to be involved in their care and in healthcare decisions made about them. According to Menzies Lyth, the degree of intimacy that would come with person-oriented care would bring with it the fear of being overwhelmed by sharing in the suffering of patients.

Morgan (1997), another organisational theorist, provides a framework to help us understand the ways in which healthcare organisations may defend themselves against the guilt that would arise if they honestly admitted that they were task- rather than patient-oriented. According to Morgan, organisations often protect themselves by using 'defence mechanisms'. At an individual level, defence mechanisms refer to the ways in which individuals defend themselves against blame and guilt. Morgan argues that these can occur in a larger scale at the level of the socially constructed organisation. A common organisational defence mechanism is 'rationalisation'.

ACTIVITY 2.9   PRACTICAL

Conduct an informal survey (i.e. ask around) among ward nurses about what prevents them spending more time with their patients/clients and talking with/listening to them. Make a note of the kinds of answers you get and share them in your class. What are the **rationalisations** given in the answer?

You will find possible answers to this activity at the end of the chapter.

Busyness affecting group and individual behaviour

'We're too busy' is a much-voiced reason given for why nurses often don't find the time simply to be with their patients, as opposed to doing nursing tasks. There may be some truth in this assertion in circumstances where there are staff shortages. However, a basic understanding of the ways in which nurses and other healthcare staff think and behave in groups (Augoustinous et al., 2006) may help us better understand the organisational social process by which clients' communication and interpersonal needs are either often ignored or treated as an irritant. This may especially be the case if these needs are seen by staff to conflict with the real business of the healthcare setting.

Augoustinous and her social psychologist colleagues describe the various ways in which patients, who seek attention from nursing staff, often for very good reasons, may be negatively 'labelled' in these circumstances. The kinds of mindsets that develop in nursing workgroups in any discipline are often very defensive and, complementary to Menzies Lyth's and Morgan's theorising, serve an anxiety reduction function.

These mindsets may take the form of 'them and us' thinking, where 'us' is viewed as reasonable and hardworking and 'them' as manipulative and troublesome. Unfortunately, 'them and us' thinking is associated with the production of irrational **prejudice** based on often insufficiently informed first impressions, with a failure to correctly and fairly read patients and clients at either empathic or theory of mind levels.

Belonging to the group or standing up for the patient?

In ending this chapter, we invite student nurses to engage in a challenge. This is to recognise when the above kinds of healthcare group processes are happening to the disadvantage of the communication and interpersonal needs of their patients or clients, and to act appropriately. Professional ethics of nursing practice, NMC standards and the need to respond in an emotionally and empathically attuned way to your patient may pull you in one direction, while the need to retain the good opinion of the work group pulls you in the other.

ACTIVITY 2.10   REFLECTIVE

Consider how you might resolve the above dilemma.

As this activity is based on your own observations and decision-making abilities, there is no outline answer at the end of the chapter.

CHAPTER SUMMARY

This chapter has introduced you to some of the key concepts and definitions related to communication and interpersonal skills (CIPS). Two frameworks for communication have been described. The rationales for safe practice and evidenced-based care have been discussed. Concepts related to CIPS, such as suffering, healthy relating and empathy, have been introduced to give you an understanding of their importance. Such importance is particularly relevant in healthcare settings, where the careful development of sensitive helping-trusting relationships with individuals is needed – individuals who are suffering because of their potential loss of control of functions, abilities and other attributes that make them human and give them dignity.

The organisational and environmental contexts have been explored to provide a backdrop to the notion that organisational environments shape experience. Such experience has a major impact on how we behave and respond in situations, and therefore on our CIPS development.

Activities: brief outline answers

Activity 2.1 (page 28)

What is the purpose of communication in healthcare settings?

- To provide and share information.
- To promote understanding of patients' and clients' responses to health problems or adjustments to their health.
- To explain options for care and treatment to patients and clients.
- To facilitate their well-being.
- To alleviate their anxieties.

Activity 2.4 (page 31)

What are the challenges to implementing evidence-based CIPS?

- Staff may find the need to alter the ways they have practised for a long time too threatening to consider and do.
- If staff were to embrace evidence-based CIPS, it might indicate to them that what they had been doing up to now, in the name of good communication, left a lot to be desired. So, rather than face this implication, it may be better for them psychologically to ignore attempts or imperatives to change.
- Staff may not be aware of evidence-based CIPS.

Activity 2.9 (page 40)

What prevents ward nurses from spending more time with their patients/clients and talking with/listening to them?

- Staff may say that they are too busy for this to happen.
- They may also say that, if they start to spend more time with their patients/clients, then the latter might come to expect this on a regular and frequent basis.

KNOWLEDGE REVIEW

Having completed the chapter, how would you now rate your knowledge of the following topics?

	Good	Adequate	Poor
1. Why the healthy, safe and effective practice of CIPS should aspire to becoming evidence-based.			
2. The reasons why CIPS in nursing are important with regard to underpinning nursing, and related, theory.			
3. The relationship between CIPS and the bases for healthy relating.			

Where you're not confident in your knowledge of a topic, what will you do next?

Further reading

Frost, PJ, Dutton, JE, Worlen, MC and Wilson, A (2000) Narratives of compassion in organizations, in Fineman, S (ed.) *Emotion in Organizations*, 2nd edition. London: SAGE Publications.

Gilbert, P (2009) *The Compassionate Mind*. London: Constable.

Both of the above texts provide a thoroughly evidence-based approach to the development of compassion as an antidote to cold, heartless and unpleasant social relating and environments.

Useful websites

www.compassionatemind.co.uk/ Set up in 2006, The Compassionate Mind Foundation aims to promote well-being through the scientific understanding and application of compassion. We're sure you will enjoy using this excellent website.

3. Evidence-based principles

CHAPTER AIMS

After reading this chapter, you will be able to:

- understand key issues in the historical development of research in communications and interpersonal skills (CIPS) in nursing;

- describe the relationship between research in CIPS and teaching and experiential learning;

- articulate the problems around relying solely on humanistic counselling/psychotherapy models of communication;

- describe the reasons for the importance of good interpersonal and organisational climates in the practice of nursing CIPS;

- understand what is meant by patient/client first- and second-level forms of communication;

- understand what is meant by 'blip cultures' and the forms of communication appropriate to such cultures.

Introduction

This chapter will enable you to analyse and evaluate critically the literature on evidence-based communication and interpersonal skills (CIPS) that are relevant to nursing practice. First, we will address the history and development of research in interpersonal communication in nursing. We will then turn to issues around teaching and learning, and the relative success of the uptake of skilled interpersonal communication among nurses. You will hopefully see that the nursing literature in this area ignores key research and theoretical work on the importance of the context of interpersonal communication, including the organisational, or work-setting, context. From this basis, you will be able to evaluate the relative contribution of counselling and psychotherapy models of CIPS. We will argue that, while these models claim to provide useful principles for practice, they must be modified according to work-setting contexts, and must also be evaluated according to contemporary theory and research in the area of social cognition, which is the study of how people process social information (there is more on social cognition in Chapter 4).

The chapter will end with the provision for you of a set of evidence-based principles for practice, and we will also include information from conceptual, empirical and policy literature about what it means to be client/patient- and carer-centred.

The historical development of research in CIPS in nursing

The historical development of an evidence-based interest in CIPS in nursing is well documented (Macleod Clark, 1985). According to MacLeod Clark, research interest in the area developed throughout the latter half of the twentieth century and included patient satisfaction surveys; studies exploring the benefits of improved communication; observational studies that described and analysed the ways in which nurses and their patients and clients interacted; and studies on the effectiveness of interpersonal skills teaching.

Banister and Kagan (1985) argued that research work on interpersonal skills in nursing was influenced by research traditions in other fields, including sociology and social, clinical, management and counselling psychology. From these disciplines, a set of desirable skills emerged, particularly social skills, empathy and assertion training.

Thus, during the latter decades of the twentieth century, nursing interpersonal research was greatly influenced by social skills and assertion training assumptions (Davidson, 1985). It was assumed that, in order to develop and hone interpersonal skills, nurses and their patients and clients needed to be both socially skilled and assertive. This is indicated by the circular view that the interpersonally skilled nurse is defined as such by having social and assertiveness skills (and (group) facilitation skills) (Morrison and Burnard, 1991).

The relationship between research in CIPS and teaching and experiential learning

The above nursing interpersonal research, in turn, influenced assumptions around developing a 'lifelong learning' approach to acquiring interpersonal skills as a feature of professional development and **experiential learning**:

> *The most obvious methods of monitoring progress in interpersonal skills development (are) . . . practising the skills involved and . . . noticing our changing and developing reactions. The practice element often comes with the job. We are involved in interpersonal relationships every day of our professional lives so there is plenty of time for trying out new behaviour. It has to be noted, however, that the decision to try out new interpersonal behaviour must be a conscious one. It is very easy to attend a workshop on counselling skills and to believe that a lot was gained from it. The truth is of course that the workshop will only have been successful if the learning gained in it is transferred to the 'real' situation. There is always a danger of an interpersonal skills workshop being an 'island' in the middle of a busy working life – something that was interesting at the time, but of little practical value.*
>
> (Burnard, 1996, p93)

A group of busy nurses go on a communication course and learn the principles of good CIPS. They return to their ward and, after a month, the ward manager wonders why the number of complaints about poor communication hasn't gone down at all. Discuss as a group why this may be so.

Brown et al. (2006) analysed the assumption that a communication skill, once learned, can be readily transferred from one context to another. In particular, they were critical of the assumptions displayed in the work of Burnard and colleagues that communication skills, derived from counselling models that assume dedicated communication time, can reasonably be transferred to busier contexts where there is very little time available.

ACTIVITY 3.1   REFLECTIVE

Think about the various contexts within which you try to communicate effectively with your clients. What are the contextual factors that both facilitate, and limit, good communication?

As this activity is based on your own reflection, there is no outline answer at the end of the chapter.

An apparent lack of attention to the ways in which organisational contextual factors may undermine the practice of skilled interpersonal communication is shown by much of the writing on CIPS in nursing. This may have influenced continual frustration about the fact that, although skilled interpersonal communication is talked up in nurse education and literature, its practice in real-life healthcare situations leaves a lot to be desired (MacLeod Clark, 1985). Brown et al. argued that this is not really surprising, since there are clear contextual differences between what is taught and what is practised:

While practitioners may well have absorbed the professional wisdom about the importance of communication in ensuring good outcomes for clients and themselves, they may well continue using timeworn communicative strategies of the kind that lead to complaints, poor outcomes and a sense of alienation between client and practitioner.

(2006, p4)

The Hargie-Dickson model of interpersonal communication and its relevance for nursing

In contrast to writing on interpersonal communication by nurse academics, Hargie and Dickson (2004), who come from a communications rather than a nursing background, were very clear about the major role of contextual factors. Summarising and synthesising research, theory and practice in the area, these authors argued that skilled interpersonal communication can be accounted for in terms of the *person-situation context*. This means that all communication is context-bound, in that it is always embedded in time, place, the specific form of the relationship of the communicators, and the organisational frameworks within which communication takes place. The personal characteristics of the communicators, together with the above features of the shared situation, act to shape the interaction by determining the goals pursued, and the responses, feedback and perception of the communication event among all those involved. Therefore, if nursing research and teaching on interpersonal communication took greater account of the contextual factors, this may lead to improved CIPS.

Counselling/psychotherapy models of CIPS and their use in nursing

Despite the concern expressed by Brown and his colleagues about the limitations of counselling and psychotherapy models for the practice of skilled interpersonal communication, a look through the literature on CIPS relevant to nursing reveals a central assumption about the relevance of classic models of counselling and psychotherapy for nursing practice (see, for example, Brown et al., 2006; Burnard, 1996; Kagan et al., 1986; McCabe and Timmins, 2006). In recent years, this assumption has resulted in the circular argument that the interpersonally skilled nurse is one who has counselling skills (Morrison and Burnard, 1991).

Clearly, counselling and psychotherapy models have contributed greatly and have transformed nursing theory, knowledge and practice from the latter half of the twentieth century. The work of Carl Rogers (1961), for example, has influenced the shift from a task- to a person-centred and holistic view of nursing care, with specific regard to the adoption of Rogers' 'core conditions' approach to human relating (now known as the 'Rogerian' approach). Rogers identified what he claimed were three 'necessary and sufficient' conditions for helping someone change effectively through a good therapeutic relationship. These are:

- acceptance or unconditional positive regard by the nurse for the patient/client;
- the nurse's therapeutic genuineness;
- empathy.

The cognitive behavioural psychotherapeutic tradition has also brought major benefits to basic and post-basic mental health nursing practice (Duncan-Grant, 2001; Grant et al., 2004). Since the early 1970s, specialist nurse cognitive behavioural psychotherapists (for example, Duncan-Grant, 2001; Newell and Gournay, 2000) have made a major contribution to the developing theory and practice of both mental health nursing generally (Newell and Gournay, 2000) and cognitive behavioural psychotherapy specifically (Duncan-Grant, 2001).

Cognitive behavioural approaches are increasingly adopting an integrative stance (Gilbert and Leahy, 2007; Grant et al., 2008). In simple terms, this means that major theoretical and empirical developments, are being incorporated into cognitive behavioural approaches. One such empirical development, having theoretical roots in psychoanalytic psychotherapy and clear relevance for nursing practices is the concept of 'transference'.

THEORY SUMMARY

Transference

Psychotherapy theories have long suggested that the mental representations an individual holds about significant others may either facilitate or impede an individual's progress towards recovery. Significant others are individuals that we have either loved or loathed in our earlier life. A new person can be experienced as either a friend or foe in a matter of moments. In support of psychotherapy theories, and in line with contemporary developments in social cognition research, Miranda and Andersen (2007) argue that transference occurs automatically in everyday life, when representations of significant others are triggered. Transference is thus a process by which people re-experience past relationships in their everyday social relationships and interactions.

Mental representations of significant others exist in memory, and such representations can easily be triggered by relevant cues in any context. Our global view about ourselves and about significant others are linked in memory. Concurrent activation occurs: when one is activated, the other is too. Transference includes assumptions about the other's presumed feelings about oneself and vice versa, and is directly linked to the concepts of schema, prejudice and stereotyping (see pages 50–2 in this chapter and also Chapter 7).

Criticisms of counselling and psychotherapy models for interpersonal communication in nursing

It has been argued that, in spite of their benefits, the relevance of some counselling and psychotherapeutic principles for day-to-day nursing care can be criticised from several perspectives. Nurses are charged with the ability to be able to demonstrate cultural and political awareness of their societal role and related professional behaviours (see also Chapter 7). In this context, Grant (2002) has highlighted cultural and political concerns with the appropriateness of the **humanistic** approach in general. He encourages students to be engaged with the literature and debate the role that individualistic psychology, which focuses on the individual without considering societal influences such as politics and paternalism (for example, the 'nanny state'), plays in everyday healthcare practice.

In a comparison of the Rogerian approach with the view of humans as rational (individualistic) economic beings, Howard (2001) argued that Rogerian counsellors concentrate on humans as childlike beings who are not influenced by, or constrained by, the realities of the society in which they live. This society is individualistic, rather than wishing to serve the best interests of all humanity, and is constrained by materialism and 'survival of the fittest'. Thus, he was posing the idea that humanistic approaches are naive.

The main criticism to emerge is that we should be wary of a simplistic understanding and practice of **Rogerian principles**. If interpersonal communication is practised independently of the contexts that shape such communication, the differences in organisational power and status between communicators are overlooked.

Further specific criticisms of the relevance of Rogers' core conditions, and related concepts, for nursing practice include challenging the following assumptions:

- that the core conditions are indeed both necessary and sufficient;
- that non-judgementalism is indeed possible between people communicating;
- that self-awareness and empathic communication is practised successfully.

These assumptions will be scrutinised, in turn, below.

The core conditions: necessary and sufficient?

From an evidence-based psychotherapeutic perspective, it has long been recognised that, while there is agreement that the core conditions are necessary for good psychotherapeutic relationships, they are often not, in and of themselves, sufficient to help clients with mental health difficulties make changes in themselves and in their lives (see, for example, Beck et al., 1979; Thwaites and Bennett-Levy, 2007). Perhaps at this point it is important to flag up the distinction made in the previous chapter between the formal practice of counselling and psychotherapy, and the relevance of using principles deriving from them in the service of developing effective relationships with clients and patients.

Non-judgementalism

There is a crucial question that must be asked by nurses interested in the use of Rogerian core conditions for enhancing CIPS. This is: to what extent is the exercise of non-judgementalism relevant and possible in nursing practice? Based on Rogers' condition of acceptance or unconditional positive regard, humanistic practitioners and writers often advocate non-judgementalism. Burnard, for example, urges health professionals to *Try suspending judgement on other people until you fully hear what they say. Even then, try to remain non-judgemental! This skill is one of the basic pre-requisites of effective counselling* (1996, p14).

A major problem with this standpoint is that empirical work in social cognition (social thinking; see also Chapter 4) suggests that it is impossible for human beings to be non-judgemental. It seems necessary, and often helpful for all of us, to take 'cognitive shortcut' judgements to make sense of contextual situations and individuals within those (Augoustinos et al., 2006). As we grow up, we develop what are described as '**schemas**' to make sense of the world (see also Chapter 7). Schemas can be thought of as mental structures that contain general expectations and knowledge of the world. This may include general expectations about people, social roles, social events, and how to behave in specific situations (Hargie and Dickson, 2004).

THEORY SUMMARY

Different types of schema have been identified (Fiske and Taylor, 1991):

- **Self-schemas:** these have to do with knowledge of ourselves.
- **Event schemas (or scripts):** these relate to the sequence of events characterising particular, frequently encountered, situations, such as buying an item from a shop, organising a doctor's appointment, or arranging a holiday.
- **Role schemas:** these guide our expectations of how people should behave according to unspoken rules of gender, race, class, power and influence.
- **Causal schemas:** these enable us to form judgements about the relationship between cause and effect in our material and social environment, and to adopt problem-solving strategies based on these judgements.
- **Person schemas:** these enable us to make a judgement about the social categories to fit other people into.

It is useful to think of schemas lying dormant, in the sense that we are usually not always consciously aware of their influence on our emotions, thinking and behaviour. However, there are times when our personal schemas can be activated so that we are more 'in touch' with them (for example, the negatively held self-schema 'I am useless' or 'I am worthless' may be activated at times of acute stress). Equally, our personally held schemas may be violated (for example, getting into trouble over something when you believe that you've done nothing wrong and that you are a fundamentally good person). Finally, the actions of others may activate the schemas we hold about either other people generally or particular groups of people.

ACTIVITY 3.2   REFLECTIVE

Imagine that, for the first time in your life, you have been stopped by a policeman who accuses you of speeding while driving. With the different types of schemas in mind, from the theory summary box above, consider what schemas about yourself and/or others have been either activated, violated, or both.

As this activity is based on your own reflection, there is no outline answer at the end of the chapter.

The human ability to make shortcut judgements has clear advantages and disadvantages. From Activity 3.2, on the one hand, it should be realised that it is to our advantage to expect what kind of interpersonal encounter is likely to happen in situations where there are clear contextual, situational and relational cues to determine behaviour (Hargie and Dickson, 2004).

On the other hand, it is equally likely that many of us will make judgements based on prejudice-related stereotyping (Augoustinous et al., 2006; Hargie and Dickson, 2004; Oakes et al., 1994; Tourish, in Long, 1999). When we stereotype others, we place them in general categories and ignore their individual characteristics. The cost of this is that *we fail to appreciate the complete uniqueness of the whole person, ensuring that our stereotypes sometimes lead us into judgements that are both erroneous and biased* (Tourish, in Long, 1999, p193).

To be discussed and developed more in Chapter 7, it is a social fact that stereotypes are widely held about social groups and individual people. It is also clear that stereotypes can become self-fulfilling. For example, if a nurse regards all shaven-headed men as aggressive, she or he might act towards them in a defensively belligerent way, which, in turn, may well precipitate an aggressive reaction from them that confirms the nurse's stereotype.

ACTIVITY 3.3   REFLECTIVE

Take a few minutes to consider whether there are any individuals, or groups of individuals, that you have a prejudice towards. Having identified an individual or a group, consider what sources of information you are using to inform your prejudice. Equally, think about the things that you don't know about the individual or group that may have a bearing on you sustaining or dropping your prejudice about them.

As this activity is based on your own reflection, there is no outline answer at the end of the chapter.

Prejudice and related stereotyping are particularly relevant problems for interpersonal communication in nursing. As described above, if a nurse, for example, acts towards a patient/client 'as if' they were completely like the stereotype the nurse imagines, the patient is likely to respond in, possibly, a defensive or angry way, often because they are aware that they've been unjustly 'put in a box'. The patient/client's behaviour may then confirm to the nurse that their (prejudiced, stereotyping) attitude was correct and the nurse may not be sufficiently aware of the fact that they are acting towards the patient/client on the basis of unfair and inappropriate judgemental attitudes.

Given the inevitability about making instant contextual evaluations about people, and their advantages and disadvantages, it seems more reasonable for people to strive towards being more constantly and critically aware of the judgements they are making about people, rather than trying to be 'non-judgemental' in Burnard's (1996) sense. Critical awareness of such judgements can also, helpfully, contribute to their modification when nurses try to get to know the person behind the stereotype. This requires nurses to practise in a **'metacognitive'** manner (Hargie and Dickson, 2004) – in other words, to think about the ways in which they think about other people.

Self-awareness

A further question for nurses considering the viability of the humanistic approach for CIPS is: what are the threats to the nursing practice of the humanistic principle of **'self-awareness'**?

It is often argued (for example, see McCabe and Timmins, 2006) that self-awareness is a significant tool for improving nurse–patient/client interaction and should be an integral part of nurse education. In this vein, based on the inherent benefits of being self-aware, it is equally asserted that self-awareness is essential for the successful implementation of the therapeutic relationship (McCabe and Timmins, 2006). Others have flagged up the importance of its use in the professional and personal development of nurses (see, for example, Burnard, 1996; McCabe and Timmins, 2006). In a style very characteristic of such uncritical acceptance of the 'self-awareness' principle in the nursing CIPS literature, Kagan et al. (1986, 21) stated that:

> self-awareness is central to interpersonal skill. We use knowledge about ourselves to plan our part in any interaction, and to put these plans into practice: our past experience contributes to our attitudes and values and affects what we notice about other people's behaviour, and how we interpret it. Understanding our reactions to what others say and do will help us to relate more effectively to them.

Given the above, and the discussion that preceded it, it may not be unreasonable to assume that it is important to strive to be as aware as possible of our attitudes, beliefs about others and behaviour towards them. However, a fundamental problem with the self-awareness concept is in regard to assumptions of the nature of 'the self' (Holstein and Gubrium, 2000). The notion of the coherent, single and developing self belongs to the philosophical tradition, which gave rise to humanistic psychology in the mid twentieth century, and to related counselling and psychotherapeutic principles and interventions. (See Chapter 5 for further explanations of the concept of self and self-disclosure.)

However, in line with findings from social psychology (Augoustinous et al., 2006; Holstein and Gubrium, 2000), contemporary philosophy suggests that it is more useful for us to consider ourselves to be often contradictory multiple selves, rather than coherent and predictable single selves. From this perspective, each one of us is likely to act in different, sometimes surprising and contradictory ways (to both ourselves and others), in different social contexts, thus behaving and experiencing ourselves and others inconsistently over time.

The importance of sensitivity to often complex social contexts, and to the corresponding shifting experiences of self and others, has important interrelated implications for nurses who wish to practise safe and effective CIPS that adhere in a balanced way to evidence-based principles. First, nurses should try to be constantly mindful of contextual factors within which relationships with patients and clients are embedded (Hargie and Dickson, 2004), rather than inflexibly trying to adhere to a prescriptive set of communication rules and expectations of context-free and predictable selves, which, by default, will ignore contextual factors.

Second, nurses need to be mindful of the lack of context in **evidence-based practice** generally, including that which informs CIPS specifically (Brown et al., 2006; Hargie and Dickson, 2004). In this regard, McCabe and Timmins argue that:

[the use of the] principles of good communication . . . rather than nurses in the health care setting using static models of communication, results in more effective patient-centred communication . . . Several contemporary authors contend that current theories of nursing and models of nursing are inadequate to inform the complexity of healthcare situations.

(2006, 167)

Essentially, McCabe and Timmins argue against a 'one model fits all' approach to both evidence-based practice and related forms of communication and interpersonal relating. In these authors' view, nurses should always be mindful of, and respond to, the individual meaning and context of each interpersonal situation in complex shifting healthcare environments.

Activity 3.4   Reflective

Think about the different contexts within which you try to practise good, effective, communication skills with your clients/patients. In what ways do these contexts limit your communication exchange?

As this activity is based on your own reflection, there is no outline answer at the end of the chapter.

Empathy

Rogers defined empathy as occurring when:

the therapist is sensing the feelings and personal meanings which the client is experiencing in each moment, when he can perceive these from 'inside', as they seem to the client, and when he can successfully communicate something of that understanding to his client.

(1967, p62)

A shorter definition, provided by Kohut, described empathy as *the capacity to think and feel oneself into the inner life of another person* (1984, p82) (see also Chapter 2 in this book).

It seems difficult to argue against the importance for nursing of the ability to enter another person's feelings and, without losing objectivity, see the world through their eyes. However, Lauder et al. (2002) state, on the basis of the cumulative evidence from the literature, that many recipients of healthcare professional interventions, including nursing care, do not believe that professionals understand either their feelings or their perspectives. It is clear that a limited ability to identify and understand the feelings and perspectives of clients and patients may result in care that fails to meet their goals, allow them to have a part in problem solving, or result in more favourable health outcomes (Sloane, 1993; Tait, 1985).

Empathy in context

There are two important contexts for the exercise of empathy: the interpersonal context and, in related and broader terms, the organisational, or work-setting, 'interpersonal climate'.

The interpersonal context

With regard to the interpersonal context, Greenberg (2007) argues that health workers who display empathy both enable the patient/client to become self-soothing, and are more likely to create a good emotional relationship with them. In short, the health worker who conveys genuine interest, acceptance, caring, compassion and joy, and no anger, contempt, disgust or fear, creates the environment for a secure emotional bond.

The nurse's facial, postural and vocal expressions of emotion clearly set very different emotional climates. Based on evidence from neuroscience, Greenberg argues that patients' and clients' right brain hemispheres respond more to nurses' facial communication than to nurses' words. Quite simply, clients and patients learn who they are, and how acceptable they are, from the facial expressions of their nurses.

ACTIVITY 3.5   REFLECTIVE

Take a few moments to read the questions below and then try to answer them for yourself as honestly as you can.

- How comfortable are you with patients or clients expressing their feelings towards you, such as their anger or grief?
- Are there times when you feel negative feelings – for example, disgust or anger – towards your patients or clients?

- Would you rather that your clients or patients were happy, rather than sad or angry, in your presence? Why?

- How 'on duty' and available are you for the people you try to help? Do you ever find yourself drifting off into your own world?

- How comfortable are you with disclosing your feelings to your patients or clients?

- How comfortable are you about showing grief in response to another's grief?

Look at yourself in a mirror and imagine yourself to be in any of the six situations listed above and move your face into an expression that you think you would have in different interactions with patients. Assess for yourself whether you look genuine, comfortable, masklike, disrespectful or disinterested.

As this activity is based on your own reflection (literally, this time!), there is no outline answer at the end of the chapter.

The organisational climate

Based on a review of the literature, and theoretical and empirical work, Reynolds and Scott (1999) contextually locate empathy in the interpersonal climate of the healthcare setting. Patients need to feel safe in their relationships and this depends on the development of trust. In these authors' judgement, trust in this context depends on the promotion of a culture of warmth and genuineness, in which disclosure and non-judgemental exploration of experiences and feelings can occur. This highlights the importance of the evidence-based need to look at the organisational conditions influencing and determining the form and content of interpersonal communication in nursing.

From this basis, it might be reasonable to pose the question: what happens when the interpersonal context and climate work against the development and practice of empathy? Supporting the contemporary work on social cognition discussed earlier, in particular the exercise of the five types of schema (self, event, role, causal and person) and stereotyping, Rogers (1961) argued that a barrier to exploration of feelings is a very natural tendency to evaluate, disapprove and judge, especially when a patient/client's communication is ambiguous or threatening. In these circumstances, nurses can become:

> *defensive, often transmitting this to the client through unwanted advice, failure to respond to direct questions, or curt unfriendly voice tone . . . [according to Rogers. . .] the logical means of correcting this tendency is to work on achieving genuineness . . . once this is established, the work of helping proceeds through the helper's moment-by-moment empathic grasp of the meaning and significance of the client's world.*
>
> (Reynolds and Scott, 2000, p229)

ACTIVITY 3.6   **REFLECTIVE**

Consider the things that get in the way of you both experiencing, and practising, empathy with your patients/clients on a day-to-day basis at work.

As this activity is based on your own reflection, there is no outline answer at the end of the chapter.

RESEARCH SUMMARY

Work on achieving genuineness in order to enhance a nurse's ability to be empathic begs the question of how empathy is taught. Based on a review of the literature, Reynolds et al. (1999) argued that empathy training in nurse education is limited by a failure to define empathy specifically and to locate it within an interpersonal theory. They also asserted that a further problem for empathy education was related to its value for the realities of clinical practice. Reynolds and his colleagues concluded that there is a need for new ways of helping nurses to develop their abilities to express empathy in clinical contexts because of the low levels of empathy in nursing and the limitations of existing empathy courses. Among other conclusions from the literature reviewed, they highlighted that:

- the optimum length of an empathy course is unclear;
- there is no common agreement about which components of an empathy course are effective;
- it is unclear what the long-term consequences of empathy training are for nurse–patient relationships;
- empathy education needs to have relevance to the clinical circumstances in which it really matters;
- therefore, clinically focused education may provide nurses with a more meaningful development of empathy skills.

Patient/client first- and second-level forms of communication

Of relevance to the argument for nurses so far is the work of Morse et al. (1992). Morse and her colleagues discussed the differences between nurses behaving in a client/patient-focused or **nurse-focused** way and whether the communication was spontaneous (which Morse called 'first level') or learned (termed 'second level).

According to these authors, client/patient-focused, first-level communication is emotionally driven and culturally conditioned and, therefore, is often an unconscious response on the part of the nurse. This type of communication includes responses such as pity, sympathy, consolation, compassion, commiseration and reflexive reassurance. This is often regarded as normal, everyday communication, but is often undervalued and seen as superficial.

Patient-focused, second-level (learned) communication includes responses such as sharing self, confronting, comforting, humour and informative reassurance. This is an important form of communication, but it is important that the interaction is, relatively speaking, focused on the client/patient rather than the nurse (although nurses, of course, do have to give some information on themselves).

Nurse-focused, first-level responses include guarding, dehumanising, withdrawing, distancing, labelling and denying, often rationalised within the 'busy nurse' persona (see Chapter 2 of this book). Deriving in large part from the work of Menzies Lyth (1988), these can be conscious or unconscious responses that nurses use to detach from difficult or emotionally demanding situations in order to cope with stress or very intense feelings. This results in task- rather than patient/client-focused work, which tends to isolate patients/clients, making them feel more anxious and lonely. Along with task-focused work comes a reduction in good CIPS.

Nurse-focused, second-level communication includes rote or mechanical responses, false pity and false reassurance. Nurses who communicate in this way can appear distant and uncaring to their patients or clients, making them feel undervalued. This, in turn, lowers the self-esteem of patients and clients (Fennell, 1999) and may undermine the trust that they have for nurses and their willingness to talk with nurses about how they are feeling, either physically or psychologically.

This level of communication is characterised by conversation closure statements on the part of the nurses, such as 'don't worry' and 'everything will be fine'. Patients and clients may thus begin to believe that they are over-reacting to their own illnesses. On the nurses' part, consciously or unconsciously (Menzies Lyth, 1988), they may use this form of communication to prevent patients or clients from verbalising any further fears. At a conscious level, this may be done because nurses genuinely feel that they don't have the time to listen. However, at an unconscious level, conversation closure behaviour on the part of nurses may mean that the emotions behind their patients' or clients' questions are too intense to deal with.

ACTIVITY 3.7   REFLECTIVE

With the above discussion and framework of first- and second-level communication in mind, keep an eye out in your practice areas for closure forms of communication. What do you think the factors at play might be in nurses demonstrating such communication?

As this activity is based on your own reflection, there is no outline answer at the end of the chapter.

Organisational environmental threats to interpersonal nursing interventions

From an environmental perspective, you can see from the discussion so far that settings that nurses work in often do not lend themselves to the time, consistency and effort required to support clients and patients with CIPS based on counselling or psychotherapeutic interventions, for three main interrelated reasons.

First, it has long been recognised in the literature of organisational theory that, in spite of claims to the contrary by particular organisations, their members may be socialised into tacitly held rules of the organisation that favour custom, practice and tradition, and are thus antagonistic to the uptake and development of evidence-based approaches (Duncan-Grant, 2001; Pfeffer, 1981).

Second, the kind of counselling intervention approaches favoured by advocates of Rogerian principles have often been criticised on the grounds of 'naive humanism'. This means that simply trying to create the facilities of empathy, unconditional positive regard and congruence between staff members, and between staff and patients or clients, is unlikely to lead to the level of effective and good CIPS desired by staff. This is because real or perceived organisational imperatives, such as busyness, lack of time or technical tasks, are likely to get in the way (Brown et al., 2006). Because of such organisational rules, custom, practice and imperatives, and because of broader trends in contemporary society favouring brief communication, Brown and his colleagues argue that counselling and psychotherapy-based communication and interpersonal models have become increasingly old-fashioned.

Blip culture communication

Brown et al. (2006) argue that we live in a time they describe as characterised by **'blip culture'** forms of interpersonally relating. This means that the leisurely conversations of the past (if such a time ever existed for nurses) were possible only because the organisational context of nursing practice allowed for this. In their view, blip culture health organisational members now only have time for brief interpersonal exchanges with their clients and patients. The challenge for nurses is in making these brief exchanges effective and empathic in the light of the preceding discussion.

Concluding remarks: implications for nursing practice

In conclusion, the following interrelated set of evidence-based principles for the increasingly skilled practice of interpersonal communication has emerged from the preceding discussion.

- Nurses would do well to consider the limitations of a sole investment in humanistic, counselling models of CIPS. A more empirically sound approach suggests that the person-situation context of communication is crucial.
- Metacognitive practice by nurses (or thinking about how they think about the ways in which they communicate and interpersonally relate to their patients or clients)

will enable exploration of the way they think about client groups and how such styles of thinking came about. This may include the personal characteristics of communication, such as self, event, role, causal or person schemas; or stereotyping; or unconsciously driven defences against intimacy with clients; or first- and second-level forms of communication. Equally, it may relate to characteristics of the organisational frameworks within which communication takes place.

- Metacognitive practice by nurses is also necessary because of the way they may have been socialised into particular organisational communication styles, which may in turn either enhance or pose a threat to skilled interpersonal practice.

- Given the principle that all communication is governed by context, although – usually unlikely – some environments may lend themselves to leisurely interpersonal exchanges, others are more appropriate for brief, 'blip culture' forms of communication. Equally, some organisational contexts may promote ineffective, damaging or abusive types of communication.

- From the basis of the above principles, it will be useful for nurses to practice the specifics of empathy. This includes empathy both in the interpersonal context and in the work-setting, or interpersonal climate, context. To facilitate this, clinically focused empathy education is relevant and much needed.

CHAPTER SUMMARY

This chapter has introduced you to the idea that there are key issues in the historical development of research in CIPS in nursing. Specifically, there is a clear relationship between research in CIPS and teaching and experiential learning. Nurses may give a variety of reasons for spending insufficient time with their clients or patients. Some of these reasons will constitute rationalisations. All communication is governed by context. There are problems in nurses having a sole reliance on humanistic counselling/psychotherapy models of communication. 'Schema'-driven and schema-activated behaviour is relevant to the practice of good CIPS in nursing. Also, good interpersonal and organisational climates are relevant for the practice of good nursing CIPS. An understanding of what is meant by patient/client first- and second-level forms of communication is important for nurses. You should be able to demonstrate an understanding of the organisational environmental threats to counselling and psychotherapy nursing interventions. Finally, nurses should understand what is meant by 'blip cultures' and the forms of communication appropriate to such cultures.

Activities: brief outline answers

As the results of all the activities in this chapter are based on your own observations and decision-making abilities, there are no outline answers for this chapter.

KNOWLEDGE REVIEW

Having completed the chapter, how would you now rate your knowledge of the following topics?

	Good	Adequate	Poor
1. The understanding that all communication is governed by context.			
2. What the term 'schema' means.			
3. What first- and second-level forms of communication are.			

Where you're not confident in your knowledge of a topic, what will you do next?

Further reading

Augoustinos, M, Walker, I and Donaghue, N (2006) *Social Cognition: An integrated introduction*, 2nd edition. London: SAGE Publications.
This book will provide you with contemporary evidence-based information on social cognition, and its relationship with social identity and communication.

Brown, B, Crawford, P and Carter, R (2006) *Evidence-based Health Communication*. Maidenhead: Open University Press and McGraw-Hill Education.
This book offers a critical evaluation of the kinds of evidence that have been collected concerning both effective communication and the training health professionals receive in communication.

Useful website

www.indiana.edu/~soccog/scarch.html This is the website of the Social Cognition Paper Archive and Information Center of Indiana University. There are lots of downloads and links that will interest readers accessing this site. It is an excellent website for link access to papers and homepages on the comprehensive range of social cognition, including non-verbal communication.

4. Safe and effective practice

CHAPTER AIMS

After reading this chapter, you will be able to:

- understand the importance and relevance of a process for communicating safely and effectively;

- appreciate the need to explore hidden areas of interpersonal communication in a safe manner with examples of techniques to draw upon;

- identify and describe techniques to develop a communication relationship process and compare models for a helping relationship.

Introduction

It is generally agreed that communication and interpersonal skills (CIPS) underpin an effective and safe nurse–patient relationship. In order to understand the nature of nurse–patient relationships, it is valuable to take time to appreciate the spectrum of the different forms of relationship that occur within nurses' professional lives. For example, relationships can range from providing total physical and tangible care in extreme cases of physical illness, to emotional support of an entirely invisible nature or support through, for example, professional/social encounters in a community setting. The nature of these encounters is as varied as a colour palette and different nurses in different settings, such as caring for adults or children, in mental health settings or with clients with learning disabilities, may experience more or less of one particular area of the palette. But, in all likelihood, there will be elements of this palette in all your interpersonal relationships with patients.

Knowing how to respond and react in these many situations can be bewildering if you have to imagine how you will manage these different forms of relationships in order to be effective. This chapter aims to provide a guide in these situations to give you confidence as well as create a sense of self-awareness. This is a crucial ingredient of a safe and effective nurse–patient relationship. We will explore what it means to be safe and begin by examining some of the theory behind the way we think in social situations and how that influences how we behave. Called the **'social thinking'** processes, these are the hidden thought processes by which people process and interpret information from and about themselves (their intrapersonal world) and other persons (their interpersonal world).

The roles we take on in relationships and the phases of the nurse–patient relationship play a large part in achieving a clear and effective communication process. This chapter will explore the many roles you have within and beyond the professional settings. The fundamental core general skills that are needed in CIPS will be explained and demonstrated in practical, work-based contexts. The chapter concludes by discussing the phases of the nurse–patient relationship and by comparing two models. There is a discussion on the nature of the helping relationship in nursing and the notion that this relationship can have a therapeutic effect. The patient's role in decision making in the nurse–patient relationship is analysed in respect of recent health policy.

What does being safe mean?

'Being safe' is a term used to describe how nurse–patient relationships can be conducted without either party being harmed. Our professional duty is to ensure that patients are safe and the NMC *Code of Professional Conduct* states:

> *You have a duty of care at all times and people must be able to trust you with their lives and health. To justify that, you must:*
> - *make the care of people your first concern, treating them as individuals and respecting their dignity;*
> - *work with others to protect and promote the health and well-being of those in your care, their families and carers, and the wider community;*
> - *provide high standards of practice and care at all times;*
> - *be open and honest, act with integrity and uphold the reputation of your profession.*
>
> (Adapted from NMC, 2004b)

The key words in this opening extract from the *Code* are to protect and promote the health and well-being of patients. To achieve that, we have to be mindful that, in our communication and interpersonal relationships with patients, we are unlikely to cause harm, injury or damage. How can we do that with words, you may be saying? Well, as we know, words are powerful objects that shape the messages we are sending. How we interpret the messages is where the damage may start.

The interpretation of the meanings of words varies from person to person. In addition to this, in healthcare we are dealing with many words that are unfamiliar to patients until they have understood and learned their meaning. This applies to the names of conditions as well as the phrases and abbreviations we use as short cuts to describe objects, processes, procedures and situations.

The way in which we transmit the words in our messages can be influenced by many factors (as discussed in Chapter 2), which have to be interpreted and assimilated by both parties in the interaction. Our body language and non-verbal signals can all lead to misunderstanding and confusion if they are not correctly understood by the patient. This is further complicated by the anxiety the patient may have about their health, their previous experiences of healthcare and the relative success of those experiences, their cultural or personalised view of the world and the degree of discomfort or pain they may be experiencing during the communication. These are the distracting stimuli described by Bateson (1979) in the circular model of communication.

It is not only the interpretation the patient may place on the messages that is important. You, as a nurse, need to interpret the patient's responses correctly, so that you know how much they understand about the situation and are sure that they have understood what you are saying or are intending to do. Your interpretation is therefore equally relevant.

SCENARIO

Scenario 1

The pattern goes like this:

→ The nurse tells the patient that he must have a shower at 6 in preparation for a surgical procedure. The patient is to undergo a routine procedure and has no major health problems.

→ The patient nods, indicating he has understood. The patient has interpreted this as taking a shower at 6 p.m., whereas the nurse meant 6 a.m. So this is a semi-correct interpretation of the message. The patient is conscious of his health and keeps himself fit and well; however, he is frightened of falling in the shower and does not have a shower at home. At home he has a seat in the bath and uses a shower attachment. The nurse looks very busy and the patient does not want to be a nuisance, so he does not ask for clarification. The patient is worried about the surgery and has not slept well, so his receptivity of information is compromised by tiredness and anxiety.

→ Because the patient nodded in apparent agreement, the nurse says something like 'That's OK then' and goes to the next patient.

It's not difficult to anticipate what will happen next. The patient will not have the shower at the correct time. If the nurse does spot this in time, the patient will take a long time because he is nervous of falling in the shower; he may even fall because he is unaccustomed to using a shower. The surgery is delayed; the operating theatre's schedule is put back, causing inconvenience to patients and staff alike. If the patient were to fall, the surgery would probably be cancelled and the patient would suffer more, in addition to suffering the delayed solution to their original problem.

Let's try it again.

Scenario 2

→ The nurse tells the patient that he has to prepare for surgery (this tells the patient what the communication is all about) that morning (this tells the patient when it is going to happen). The patient needs to have a shower at 6 a.m. (it might seem obvious to state the time as this communication is taking place in the morning, but it makes it clearer and reinforces the time-frame for the patient).

→ The nurse asks the patient if he is comfortable having a shower or is there any other way that he usually has a full wash. (This gives the patient the opportunity to express his personal hygiene methods and confirm that he can shower or describe what he needs to do.)

→ The patient responds by explaining how he usually washes.

→ The nurse needs to find out not only how, but why, the patient washes in this manner, as this can shed light on any fear of falling.

→ The nurse explores how the facilities on the ward can be adapted to suit the patient and checks out if the patient agrees. As the environment is unfamiliar to the patient and his usual routine is disrupted, it would be additionally helpful if the nurse were to take the patient to the shower facilities and demonstrate to the patient how to use the shower.

During this encounter, the nurse can explore with the patient any concerns or anxieties he may have about the preparations for surgery, such as falling in the shower, and at the same time clarify any fears about the surgical procedure if these have not already been elicited during the assessment processes. This takes additional time, but could avoid a great deal of future inconvenience and potential safety issues. It could also provide opportunities to develop the nurse's relationship with the patient and understand his needs at this point in time, as well as provide preparation for their communication post-operatively.

The scenarios illustrate how a simple communication request can involve several aspects of meeting physical and emotional needs. The success of managing these aspects is often due to our abilities to perceive and interpret information. This has been studied in a branch of social psychology termed 'social cognition' and is often referred to as 'social thinking'. The aim of these studies is to find out how people take in information and assimilate it so that it can be used effectively in social situations with friends and family, but the studies can also be used to improve professional relationships.

The process of social thinking

Social thinking is the process by which people assimilate and interpret information or thoughts from and about themselves (their intrapersonal world) and other persons (their interpersonal world). Most of the time our social thinking activities work very well for us in social situations. We pay attention to the most, rather than the least, important aspects of our environment, which keeps us safe. We think about people in a way that organises our ideas into categories, so that we can recognise characteristics about people. Humans use a process of social comparison to do this. By comparing what we are encountering with what we have encountered before gives us a frame of reference or benchmark to make judgements. We can also take in all manner of facts, which originate from different sources and experiences, and organise them into categories so that we can recognise them again. Generally, we remember what we need to remember, and make conclusions about facts and ideas, all of which influences how we react and respond in situations.

Finding out more about how social thinking operates is one way to ensure we accurately understand and interpret what people around us are expressing. There is a 'recipe' for social thinking that has been built up around two of the commonest types of reaction to people and events. These are *spontaneous* and *deliberative*.

Spontaneous means 'off the top of your head' responses, such as 'all experts must be right' or 'all exotic food must taste disgusting'. These quick responses mean that we have not taken the time to gather further information or evidence to verify the judgement.

At other times, people will engage in a more deliberative response, taking time to elaborate on the statement or follow different ideas that reach away from the original thought to engage with new ideas. This comes with an analysis of problems or wider impressions of a situation or context. It is where old habitual patterns of response or assumptions are reconsidered and delved into more deeply to arrive at a fuller picture of events, ideas and impressions. Based on the work of Wyer and Srull (1986), a recipe for social thinking has been designed that describes these two stages of a process that assembles impressions, conclusions, decisions and intentions.

STAGE 1 – SPONTANEOUS

TAKE	➡	raw sensations such as sights, sounds, words and sentences
ADD	➡	these together to form an initial comprehension
ORGANISE	➡	without being aware of the decisions into handy, familiar categories
INTEGRATE	➡	with whatever you happen to be thinking of at the time
GENERATE	➡	new thoughts, which are organised and integrated with the original information.

These actions are undertaken as quickly and as automatically as possible and could be the final impression, conclusion, decision or intention. Often this is as far as people get in the recipe, because it is a quick and easy method. If, on the one hand, the topic is not important, or they have other more pressing things to do, or they are not particularly close to the person or persons involved in the situation, the process stops here.

If, on the other hand, they are more interested, are closely involved in the outcome of the situation or committed in some way – that is, more willing and able to do so – they will progress to the second stage of the process.

STAGE 2 – DELIBERATIVE

USING	➡	your current goals or aims, what you want to achieve in the situation

APPLY	➡	your general world-view knowledge, schemas from your personal previous experiences or underpinning research evidence
APPLY	➡	your knowledge of people's expectations of what they want to achieve and how they would go about it in this situation
APPLY	➡	your knowledge of the specific individuals, groups, communities and other situations such as this one that you may not have experienced personally.

There is no order in applying these deliberations; they are merely different types of knowledge that you can draw upon to assimilate information about a patient. The finished product of these deliberations is a final summary of impressions, conclusions, decisions or intentions. This may confirm an initial impression; however, it may be adjusted or altered from the initial view. The process of deeper analysis does not have to take a long time, but gathering together additional information upon which to make a judgement can provide a safer and more informed way to proceed in a nurse–patient relationship that is not based solely upon initial judgements.

Cognitive stores

Students are often surprised that experienced staff can draw conclusions about complex situations or seem to have an intuitive understanding of patients' needs, without the patients appearing to have directly expressed those needs. One explanation for this is that experienced staff have a store of previous experiences, knowledge of different societal groups and up-to-date knowledge of contemporary research that they synthesise rapidly to form their conclusions. Their spontaneous recipe works for them. However, even the most experienced staff have occasions when they have to reflect on their judgements to ensure that they are not using habitual stereotypes or outdated research to make their decisions.

Cognitive misers

If staff do not use their cognitive stores effectively, they run the risk of becoming 'cognitive misers'. A cognitive miser is someone who does not put effort into thinking around the problem or situation, and only uses the minimum cognitive resources they need. A consequence of this is that some knowledge becomes so automatic that it is incorporated into the organising part of the recipe without any extra effort ever being put into the deliberative stage. Vital information could be overlooked.

Recency

Another danger is the recency with which a category has been used. The more recently a category is used, the more likely it is that it will be used again. The consequence of this is that new information could be consigned to the same category, when there may be differences that are relevant to consider. This can also apply to the three types of knowledge in the deliberative stage. Combining the recency factor with the cognitive miser factor means that people will not consider other options and will stop with a 'good enough' fit.

Self-generating thoughts

One final principle to discuss is how we self-generate our thoughts in the final part of the spontaneous recipe stage and the pitfalls this may provide. Even when we are tired, we generate thoughts. Our brains continue to run along by themselves even when we are in a darkened room and have little information to receive, such as the raw sensations of light, touch, heat, cold, etc. These are self-generated thoughts that flit from one topic to another, but are organised insofar as they are recognisable to us as we compare them to the knowledge categories we have established. These thoughts are not entirely random, as they are linked to significant topics that have been thought about recently (the recency factor again) and thus can be biased towards these topics. These thoughts can also become organised and integrated into familiar categories.

We can also generate scenarios that are figments of our imagination and our difficulty is that we cannot always distinguish between these and the information that is drawn from the raw sensations in the first stage of the recipe. For example, we cannot always remember whether we put the keys in their usual place or whether we imagined we did! In the same way, we cannot always differentiate between self-generated imaginings and information from actual situations. This is because the processing of the information is rapid, familiar and unconscious.

To guard against this human foible in healthcare, we need to use both spontaneous and deliberative stages in appropriate situations. When a snap judgement is required and time is not available, we make spontaneous decisions. However, to be safe and to fully understand and interpret our patients' needs, we need to communicate with them to gather information in the spontaneous stage that we can then feed into the deliberative stage. The summary from the first stage is combined with different types of knowledge in the second stage to make an informed assessment of the patients' understanding of how their health needs can be met.

ACTIVITY 4.1   REFLECTIVE

The scenarios 1 and 2 above are examples of stages 1 and 2 of the recipe. Take a moment to reflect on a conversation you have recently had with a patient/client in a recent clinical placement. Jot down the conversation. Analyse it to see if you were making decisions based upon the spontaneous or deliberative stage of social thinking.

Concentrating on the deliberative stage, what other information did you have or would you need to gather to give you a more comprehensive set of information to understand that patient's needs?

Think about where you would find further information. Would it be from research or from your knowledge of social situations or societal groups and communities?

Has it occurred to you that you can assimilate this information to help you plan your care of this patient without asking the patient a direct question?

There are further comments on this activity at the end of the chapter.

Most nurse–patient interactions are like social interactions in that they will be dynamic, creative, responsive and usually socially constructed. The primary mode of communication is talk enhanced with gestures, personal communication style and body language. This enables the two partners to exchange information, agree decisions, and develop and maintain the relationship. However, most healthcare encounters can be thought of as an interaction between two distinct cultures (Edelman, 2000) – the medical culture and the culture of the patient. The differences between the two groups are that they think differently about health and illness, and that they have different perceptions, attitudes, types of knowledge, sources of knowledge and agendas. The patients' agendas will be based upon their expectations and experiences of illness, health, consultation and treatments, whereas the healthcare professional is likely to reflect their own (usually Western) medical or health-related training together with personal background factors. Reconciling these differences is one of the major challenges to engaging in a successful nurse–patient relationship.

One way to clarify and negotiate through this conjunction of cultures is to identify in nurse–patient interactions two basic goals: either associated with information giving and responding to questions, or relationship building, which is geared towards socio-emotional gains. Separating out these goals within interactions can help clarify what will be gained from the interaction. Information giving and responding to question activities are related to adherence, or following instructions, and remembering information, whereas patient satisfaction is related to the socio-emotional aspects of interactions. Despite our best efforts at good communication, patients report the highest levels of dissatisfaction over poor communication in clinical settings (Caris-Verhallen et al., 1999).

For the nurse, there may be a desire for the patient to achieve a satisfactory understanding of procedures and processes, whereas the patient may wish to have satisfaction from receiving kindness, empathy and a sense of respect. Alternatively, patients may want information and nurses may want recognition for the work they are doing. Achieving a balance in reaching these respective goals is needed. The responsibility for understanding the balance lies with the nurse, which is why differentiating between the professional relationship and the social relationship is necessary. This is discussed further in the following chapter.

Roles

We all have several roles; some examples are daughter, brother, friend, companion, partner, parent, colleague, manager and subordinate. How many roles do you have? They all require different identities and yet they are often linked. There are occasions when roles can overlap and, in some cases, form parts of, or belong to, a particular social identity. In general, you will have a primary role and several secondary roles. In nursing, to maintain a social identity as a nurse requires acceptance, and an ability to relate to other nurses. Yet within nursing there are other specialties that involve different types of relationship. For example, critical care nurses relate in a different way to their patients in comparison with mental health nurses and their clients. The context and requirements of the roles are different. But that is not to say that critical care nurses do not relate to emotional issues (for example, see Peel (2003), who discusses breaking bad news to relatives on critical care units) or dealing with emergency mental health conditions (for example, see Broadbent et al. (2002), who devised a triage assessment tool specifically to deal with mental health emergencies in a unit where 2.6 per cent of all admissions had primary mental health issues).

ACTIVITY 4.2   REFLECTIVE

Draw a network diagram of your roles (see example below).

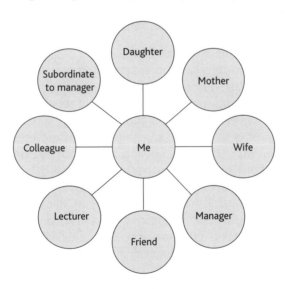

- Which are primary and secondary roles?
- Which role do you think defines you the most?

The literature suggests that social roles (i.e. roles that require taking on role-appropriate behaviours defined by rules and relationships) are where we take on a social identity but where this identity may not be our defining identity.

There are times when you may feel a conflict between roles that you have; such as being a student, which is a childlike role, and yet being beyond childhood, which is an adult role. Understanding this concept and maintaining a sense of self-identity when we are in challenging professional roles (for example, are you feeling like a nurse or a parent in a situation?) can help to manage role confusion and blurring of roles. So your answer to which role defines you most should be that your primary role may be influenced by one of your secondary roles, but the real you will be a unique and separate set of characteristics.

Now draw a diagram of a clinical placement you were in recently and include all the roles you observed there. Identify what characteristics, rules and expectations define those roles – not forgetting the patient in this analysis.

- How much does clothing define the role? Or hierarchies of responsibilities?
- Are there traditions, rituals, myths and legends associated with the roles?
- Where are role boundaries traversed? Is this safe practice?

Discuss your thoughts and answers on these questions with your fellow students.

As this activity is based on your own reflection, there is no outline answer at the end of the chapter.

Phases of the nurse–patient relationship

While there are no specific rules to guide the formation or stages of relationships, we can see from our previous discussions that various cultures, societies and groups have norms that guide how relationships and roles within those relationships should be conducted. In a healthcare setting a slightly different set of rules applies and the roles are going to be slightly different from those in a social setting. The main reason for this is that the purpose is not social, but professional. The rate at which the relationship is formed will also be different and determined by different settings. In a pre-assessment surgical assessment unit you may have only 30 minutes, whereas on a medical ward a patient may stay for a number of days. Children may have short or long periods of time in hospital. In mental health settings there will be longer time frames within which to build in-depth relationships, and in community settings the context of being in the patients' own homes provides a different pace for the stages of relationships to develop. In residential settings with learning disability clients relationships have an even longer time span in which to develop. In Chapter 1 we explored an overarching framework for CIPS. We will now look at two examples of specific relationship models.

Six-stage model of relationship formation

There will be uniformity to the phases of the relationship that can be mapped on to a six-stage model proposed by DeVito (2007). Having such a model in mind enables the nurse and patient to see how the relationship will develop and will give the purpose of the interaction, be it over a long or short period of time, a structure. Having a structure gives both nurse and patient greater clarity and can reduce confusion over how long a relationship should last and what might be expected at each stage of the relationship. The stages are *contact, involvement, intimacy* and *deterioration*, which can then lead to either *repair* or *dissolution*.

In the first stage, there is perceptual contact during which first impressions are made. Physical appearance, friendliness, warmth and openness are noted. This quickly leads into interactional contact during which opening words are offered in the form of a welcome or greeting and involve ordinary conversation. Burnard (2003) has called these openings *phatic conversations*, where ordinary conversation enhances social fellowship and small talk helps to ease situations and develop rapport with patients. Your demeanour and style set the tone for this and future conversations. Involvement is where a sense of connection and mutuality are established. Questions and answers are exchanged to establish likes and similarities or the reasons for being in a situation. Intimacy, in social settings, is where friendships, companionship and loving relationships are formed. In a **professional relationship** this is where closeness and levels of appropriate touch and deeper emotional connectedness through empathy and understanding are experienced. In Watson's (1988) transpersonal theory of nursing, she suggests that nurses can become so close to patients that they experience a kind of presencing or 'being with' patients. This can happen in circumstances when patients are dying or in the extreme stages of illness.

The deterioration phase of the model is when the parties disengage and the end of the relationship is ahead. In the professional sense this is where patients are preparing to be discharged from care and they may reduce conversations or not explore their healthcare questions with such frequency. This is an inevitable phase of the nurse–patient relationship. If patients are tending towards overdependency in the relationship, steps have to be taken to alter the intimacy of the interactions so that the patient grows accustomed to the withdrawal of contact. If patients return to the ward or unit, a process of relationship repair takes place and participants go back to a previous stage and work forwards again. The final stage is relationship dissolution and will involve patients being discharged from care or, in some cases, the death of a patient. Because of the levels of intimacy a nurse can experience through these stages, managing the closeness and remaining emotionally intact can pose challenges even to the most experienced nurse.

It is worth mentioning that these stages are not only relevant to nurse–patient relationships. Nurses are also in contact with patients' relatives, friends and carers. Often the nurse will establish a relationship with persons close to the patient that will go through similar stages, and a marginally different relationship will emerge. The relationship will be tailored to meet the requirements of those relationships yet remain professional, with a similar purpose, which is to return the patient to health, or maintain or promote health. This distinguishes these relationships from **social relationships**.

THEORY SUMMARY

Transpersonal theory of caring

Watson's theory of transpersonal caring (Watson, 1988; Watson and Foster, 2003) is useful to consider in this context. It is organised around concepts such as transpersonalism, phenomenology, the self and the caring occasion, with ten curative factors that guide nursing care. The theory is intended to encompass the whole of nursing; however, it places most emphasis on the experiential, interpersonal processes between the caregiver and recipient. It focuses on caring as a therapeutic relationship and attempts to reduce the components of caring to describable parts, so that these parts can be understood and learned. As such, the theory could be criticised for being reductionist. However, this also enables a complex phenomenon to be understood, and this is where tension exists between reductionism and explanation. The theory claims to allow for, and be open to, **existential-phenomenological** and spiritual dimensions of caring and healing that cannot be fully explained scientifically through the Western mind of modern society. More information on the theory can be obtained from the web resources found at the end of the chapter.

The helping relationship

Within the relationship stages outlined above, the nurse will engage in specific techniques to assist and help the patient. This is termed the 'therapeutic relationship'. According to Henderson (1967), this is:

> the practice of those nursing activities which have a healing effect or those which result in movement towards health or wellness.
>
> (Henderson, 1967, px)

McMahon's (1993) view is that nursing can be therapeutic. He claims that it centres on the nurse–patient relationship and involves both overt and non-visible caring techniques.

- Developing the nurse–patient relationship based upon partnership, intimacy and reciprocity.
- Manipulating the environment – from the macro organisational level, through to the meso patient environment level to the micro environment and the physical features that impact on the well-being of the patient.
- Teaching – involving patient education and information.
- Providing comfort – physical and non-physical care.
- Adopting complementary health practices – these are creative approaches to healing that are incorporated into nursing care.
- Utilising tested physical interventions – incorporating intuitive approaches to care that can be supported by inductive research approaches.

To help nurses to carry out this aspect of their relationship with patients requires a deeper level of interaction that involves not only CIPS, but an integration of their knowledge of several domains, for example physical, social and psychological. At this stage in our discussions we will be concentrating on your needs to transfer to Branch Programmes. Therefore, to enable a more accessible approach to therapeutic care, we will examine Egan's (1998) skilled helper model. This is a framework for conceptualising the helping process. The model is linked to Rogers' core conditions of genuineness, respect and empathy and provides a map for exploring relationships. It also creates an explicit set of techniques for managing relationships, as each will require individual adjustments to meet situations as they arise. There are three simple questions to answer in the model.

- What is going on?
- What do I want instead?
- How might I get to what I want?

Each of the questions relates to a stage in the model that can be followed sequentially but that may be used at any time. To answer any of the questions, the individual who is seeking answers tells their story and then explores with the helper ways to examine the options and solutions to the questions. The process involves looking at information and clarifying meanings. Early on in this chapter we talked about interpretations and perceptions and how they can exert influence. This model is a way of exploring in detail what individuals want from their healthcare and how nurses can assist them to gain the solutions they want, as well as exploring some of the realistic options to achieving better health outcomes (see 'Useful websites' at the end of the chapter for links to the model for further study).

Patients as decision makers

In 2006, the government launched the Expert Patients Programme (EPP) (DH, 2006). This was in response to the evidence that more people in the twenty-first century are living into their seventies, eighties and beyond. The implications are that patients will be living with long-term conditions and multiple pathologies. The programme is aimed at patients to enable them to self-manage their conditions and has a central tenet that patients understand their disease better than medical practitioners. That could also include nurses. Patients are seen as key decision makers in their treatment processes and this is based upon experiences and research from the UK and North America. The potential of the nurse's role in assisting the EPP is to further enable patients to find ways to solve difficulties and issues they have with their lifestyles and treatment regimes so that they can be in control. The self-management programme is run from local community centres. Nurses in acute and primary care settings can work in conjunction with this philosophy by adopting Egan's model, thus providing a framework to assist patients in decision making about their care.

ACTIVITY **4.3**   PRACTICAL

While you are on community placements, you may wish to enquire about local EPPs. On the DH website you can use a postcode to find local programmes and you may want to contact the programme organiser and meet with them to find out about how the programmes are progressing and about the role of the community nurse in relation to the programmes.

As this activity is based on your own observation, there is no outline answers at the end of the chapter.

CHAPTER SUMMARY

In this chapter we have explored the meaning of being safe without harming in interpersonal relationships in healthcare. We have also considered the relevance of social thinking models as explanatory frameworks and have explored the many roles in practice and the potential for role confusion. In addition, we have identified a process for communication and interrelationship skills in healthcare settings.

Activities: brief outline answers

Activity 4.1 (pages 67–8)

You may, however, want to verify or clarify if your judgement is correct by probing questioning. In doing this you are demonstrating to the patient that you are trying to understand their needs, that you are interested in them as a person and that you are putting effort into your professional relationship.

You are not being intrusive or asking personal questions that many patients find breach their personal boundaries. You are using your assimilated knowledge to enable effective communication.

KNOWLEDGE REVIEW

Having completed the chapter, how would you now rate your knowledge of the following topics?

	Good	Adequate	Poor
1. How social thinking impacts on your communication style.			
2. The differences between the many roles you will take in a professional setting.			
3. Evaluating the effectiveness of the six-stage model.			

Where you're not confident in your knowledge of a topic, what will you do next?

Further reading

Crawford, P, Brown, B and Bonham, P (2006) *Communication in Clinical Settings*, Foundations in Nursing and Health Care. Cheltenham: Nelson Thornes.
This is a useful book on core interpersonal skills.

Egan, EG (1998) *The Skilled Helper: A problem management approach to helping*, 6th edition. Pacific Grove, CA: Brooks Cole.
This contains a lot of information on helping relationships.

Useful websites

www.gp-training.net/training/mentoring/egan.htm A website that gives information on helping relationships.

www.nursing.ucdenver.edu/faculty/caring.htm This website has information on Watson's transpersonal theory.

5. Understanding potential barriers

Introduction

This chapter will explore those factors that may act as barriers and impede effective communication and interpersonal relationships.

First, we will investigate the shift we make in our professional work from social to professional relationships. The chapter considers how to develop safe professional relationships, by examining the different degrees of intimacy between friend and carer, and the rules of social engagement.

Next, we will consider the effect that emotions can have on communication and interpersonal relationships. Emotions are a fundamental facet of human nature and our ability to express how we feel. As such, they are a vital part of our communication methods because, when we demonstrate our emotions to our friends, family and colleagues, they can recognise how we feel and tune into our emotional needs. If only it were this simple! This seemingly straightforward aspect of interrelationships is made more complex by the need to balance our emotional expressiveness with the need to construct new ways of coping with situations and with the extent to which we express or repress our emotions. Emotions can therefore both enhance and impede communication.

Other barriers to communication will also be explored in this chapter, such as how we construct meaning and interpret communication as a function of this construction. The effect of motivation on communicating health advice is also explored.

Finally, we will consider the nature of conflict, how it is derived and techniques to diffuse conflict in healthcare situations.

Shifting from social to professional relationships

The shift from social relationships, as we know them, to professional relationships requires a transition from those we had in our early experiences or developed in our social lives that were based upon kinship or friendship networks to ones that are based upon professional values and governed by a code of practice. These values encompass a sense of purpose, mutuality, authenticity, empathy, active listening, confidentiality and a respect for the dignity of the patient/client.

This requires nurses to set aside biases, prejudices and very often their own emotions, although these very aspects of them as people are important as they bring to the encounter the humanness that is crucial to a sound professional relationship. To help you differentiate between social and professional relationships, you will see in Table 5.1 comparisons of some of the major elements of social and professional relationships. We will be exploring more of these elements as we go through the chapter.

Table 5.1: Comparison of social and professional relationships (adapted from Arnold and Boggs, 2004).

Social	Professional
• You have no specific legal or professional responsibility for the person. • You may be related or have a code of behavior that is either explicitly or implicitly agreed between a group or community that provides a framework for sanctioning different codes of behaviour. • Social engagement can be more informal in some instances and formal in others.	• A professional has the responsibility for helping the patient regain a state of health; this involves a spectrum of activities that range from the physical to the invisible. This is governed by a professional *Code of Conduct* (NMC, 2004b). • There is informality and formality in different settings and contexts. • The patient and professional have to negotiate and agree the levels of formality, some of which may be dictated by the setting, e.g. a multiprofessional case review.
• The purpose of the relationship is not necessarily specific or geared towards particular goals. • The individuals know each other through choice, social or family connections. • There is often an element of spontaneity about engaging in the relationship.	• The focus of the relationship is on the needs of the patient; often engaged through necessity rather than choice. • The behaviour of the professional will be planned, implemented and evaluated in a formal or semi-formal manner. • The participants may not know each other. • The participants may not like each other.

Table 5.1: Continued

Social	Professional
• Feelings of liking, loving or fondness are involved and often expressed. • Persons are often judgemental within the social codes of their communities or family groups about those who are beyond those groupings and may share these judgements to gain a sense of consensus in the group of group or community characteristics.	• The professional seeks to be non-judgemental and non-partisan. • Sharing of personal or intimate factors is unidirectional from the patient to the professional. • Confidentiality is a key factor in the professional relationship.
• The feelings between persons in a social relationship may enhance or may detract from the relationship course.	• The main aim of the professional is to guide and influence the patient towards a better understanding of the factors that are affecting their health and a resolution of their ill-health status. • The feelings of the patient are identified, acknowledged and accounted for in any discussions. • The feelings of the professional are woven into the encounter to respond empathetically. • Deeper personal feelings may not be appropriate to express. This is a time for careful judgement by the professional. If extreme feelings are experienced by the professional it is important to seek support from a colleague or qualified professional for guidance.
• The sense of control in the relationship is more evenly shared or driven by the wants and desires of those communicating. • The relationship may continue indefinitely or end depending on the degrees of mutual liking between the persons.	• There is usually a planned ending to the relationship as a result of the resolution to the above factors. • The professional has self- and professional knowledge through their life skills and education that are deliberately brought to bear on the encounter. • The professional takes responsibility for setting the boundaries of the relationship.

Becoming over-involved

One of the concerns professionals have is how to become involved with a patient in a sufficiently supporting manner without becoming over-involved and not being able to stand back and objectively assess the needs of the patient. Being oneself and bringing personal characteristics to the relationship is crucial, otherwise we would be very mechanical and would be like androids or robots giving care. The difference is that a professional relationship, which does indeed travel a fine line between compassion on the one hand and being so close that there is an over-involvement of emotional investment on the other, has to draw a line between the two. Becoming over-involved is most likely to happen when a nurse feels an emotional connection that reminds them of a situation from their past (see the description of transference in Chapter 3, page 48); or when there are shared feelings on a matter that can have the potential to create a strong bond.

Another source of over-involvement is when a nurse feels guilty from a previous relationship in which matters were left unresolved. This could be from either a personal or a professional experience. The nurse may attempt to resolve the issues in order to make the situation feel better than the earlier one, but the danger is that the nurse may not regard the specific needs of the patient being currently cared for. Often it will be an unconscious drive that the nurse will not be aware of. This may be noticed by others around the nurse who is transferring her feelings from a previous situation to the one that is now being experienced. It takes a very self-aware person to recognise that the feelings are related to a different situation and to set them aside so that the patient's needs become uppermost. It also takes a professionally astute colleague to recognise what is happening.

CASE STUDY

Mary is a 79-year-old woman who has severely debilitating arthritis and is cared for in a nursing home. She is a quiet, placid woman who is widowed and has five children, and although they live some distance away they do visit regularly, especially her two daughters and their children, who are now adults. Her favourite occupation is doing crossword puzzles; she is a warm and kind person who is loved by her family. Her days are long and filled with pain from her arthritis and yet her mind is still alert and she loves to converse with the nurses. She can no longer mobilise on her own and has a urinary catheter for her elimination needs, but she requires regular enemas to help evacuate her bowels as the side effects of the pain medication mean she is always constipated. She puts up with her discomforts valiantly and the nurses are noticing that she is slowly becoming sleepier each day and less interested in conversing with them. These are her twilight years.

It is very easy to become fond of Mary. She is pliant and gentle and, because she is so uncomplaining about her situation, it is easy to become attached to Mary emotionally and feel a fondness towards her. She may be like the grandma you wish you had or she may be like the grandma you had and lost. If you did not have time to say goodbye, this could be even more poignant for you. It is in this kind of situation that you have to retain your professional distance and yet still strike a balance between caring and becoming over-involved. In Chapter 1, we discussed endings and it is in a situation like this that endings need to be carefully and sensitively construed to avoid reliving previous emotional situations or experiencing regrets and guilt. Talk through your feelings with your mentor or colleagues to help you gain a sense of proportion in these situations.

Developing trusting relationships with colleagues with whom you can share your feelings about situations or relationships is a strategy that will ensure that you are being safe. Mentoring or supervision by senior staff are also effective methods for supporting staff who are dealing with complex situations where there are no simple solutions (Mullen, 2005).

Professional friend

The balance between being detached and over-involved is one that has to be finely struck. Bach (2004) found that community nurses developed a specific kind of professional relationship with their patients that they termed a '**professional friend**'. It was not a social relationship and yet it was not a detached professional relationship. This relationship was based on many of the social aspects of the relationships described above, but there did remain a fine barrier and the patients/clients always remained on one side of that line so that the professional integrity of the nurses could remain intact. This is never more apparent than when an issue arises in a relationship that requires the professional to act or respond in a way that would not challenge a friendship but would create an inevitable problem in a professional relationship. It is where codes of social behaviour are superseded by professional codes of, for example, confidentiality, or where harm is being done to another person that comes to light in the communications between professional and patient.

> Professional relationships are controlled alliances that occur within a particular context and are time limited.
>
> (Arnold and Boggs, 2004, p80)

In this sense, Arnold and Boggs are suggesting that the professional relationship is shaped by the professional because of the setting in which it is carried out. We would add that it is contingent on the needs of the patient. To establish and sustain interpersonal relationships, the nurse has to establish boundaries, or even constraints, that limit and ultimately make safe the interaction between patient and nurse in these settings. The boundaries are created from ethical, legal and professional codes of practice, as well as a patient's right to caring from nurses who appraise situations realistically in order to ensure responsive actions towards a patient's optimum health and well-being.

On the other hand, a friendship is defined as:

> An interpersonal relationship between two persons that is mutually productive and is characterized by mutual positive regard.
>
> (DeVito, 2007, p282)

There are also thought to be three friendship types:

- reciprocity, characterised by loyalty, self-sacrifice, mutual affection and generosity;
- receptivity, characterised by a comfortable and positive imbalance in the giving and receiving of rewards; each person's needs are satisfied by the exchange;
- association, a transitory relationship more like a friendly relationship than a true friendship.

Your friendships, or how you perceive friendships, will be influenced by your culture, or the type of society you inhabit, and your gender. In Middle Eastern, Asian and Latin American friendships there is an expectation that you will go out of your way to help. There is an expectation of self-sacrifice to maintain the friendship. Collectivist societies that have an emphasis on groups and communities cooperating together expect close friendship bonds to be established. However, in individualistic societies, such as in North America, you are expected to look out for yourself. Women tend towards more self-disclosure than men and men do not generally view intimate details as necessary in friendships.

ACTIVITY 5.1   PRACTICAL

Have a look at the following and mark on each line a point where you believe the statements represent either professional or social behaviours.

As the questions depend on your own findings, there is no outline answer at the end of the chapter.

	Social ————— Professional
I am happy to joke with patients	←————————→
I am always smiling whatever is happening	←————————→
I would not let a patient cry; it does no good	←————————→
I think it is best to show your feelings all of the time	←————————→
I let people tell me as much as they want me to know	←————————→
I tell people exactly what I think of them	←————————→
I let people know that there will come a time when they will leave, so that we both know what to expect	←————————→

Degrees of intimacy

When talking about intimacy in CIPS, we can be discussing two aspects. One is the physical space between persons in an interaction, which is underpinned by studies in *proxemics*. The other concerns the degree to which we disclose our inner feelings and thoughts to another, and the extent of self-disclosure required in a relationship to achieve a greater depth of intimacy in knowing and understanding between the partners. Both have relevance to understanding the relative boundaries expected in social and professional relationships.

Proxemics

Hall (1966) pioneered the study of proxemics and identified four spatial distances that also correspond to types of social relationships. They are *intimate*, *personal*, *social* and *public*.

RELATIONSHIPS AND PROXEMIC DISTANCES

Relationship	Distance
Intimate	0 — 18 inches Close — Far *Very close family and friends*
Casual-Personal	1 ————— 4 feet Close ————— Far *Informal conversations with friends and acquaintances*
Social-Consultative	4 ————— 12 feet Close ————— Far *More impersonal professional transactions*
Public	12 ————— 25 feet + Close ————— Far *Making speeches and addressing large groups at formal gatherings*

(Adapted from DeVito, 2007)

The four distances can be further divided into close and far phases. The far phase of one level can blend into the close phase of the next level. This will depend on the situation and degrees of comfort felt by individuals and also the shift from one distance to another, either to increase or contract the distance.

The theoretical explanations for these distances are conceptualised in three different ways. The first suggests that individuals hold a buffer of space around them that acts as a protection zone against unwanted attack or touching. As nursing often takes place within this zone, it is important to consider how we move into this close proximity and reduce the sense of threat that this closeness may generate. The second suggests that we strive to maintain equilibrium between varying degrees of intimacy and interpersonal relationships and that we adjust the spatial/relationship ratio accordingly. When the degree of equilibrium that you have chosen is threatened, you may make adjustments, such as avoiding eye contact on a crowded bus or turning away.

The final explanation is derived from responses where individuals find themselves having their expectations of proximity 'violated'. Called the expectancy violation theory, it holds that, in these situations, the topic of conversation becomes less important and the relationship comes into focus in its place. Those who violate expected spatial relationships are judged to be less truthful. Yet, if you are perceived positively, that is, of high status or particularly attractive, then you will be perceived even more positively if you violate the norm. If, however, you are perceived negatively and you violate the norm, you will be perceived even more negatively. It is a minefield and nurses have to tread very carefully so as not to violate the expected distance.

The way to do this is to seek permission from the patient before carrying out a personal procedure and wait for a response before continuing. This may not be possible in an emergency situation, but it is always advisable to explain to the patient what you are doing and why; even a semi-comatose person can hear a voice and this will enable the patient to be more aware of your actions. Similarly, the tone and pitch of your voice, which should be gently questioning and not commanding, will give the patient reassurance. Informing and negotiating consent to invade a patient's personal space demonstrates respect for the patient's privacy and dignity.

Self-disclosure

How much do you tell a patient about yourself to gain a sense of closeness in your professional relationship and to equalise the reciprocity between the information that you have about them versus the amount they have about you? Creating this balance is seen as a fundamental human need. First, let's consider what we may mean by 'self'. Hargie and Dickson (2004) suggest that there are nine different types of self. To help us understand these many facets, they have conceptualised these types as shown in the following box (previously discussed in Chapter 3).

TYPES OF SELF

Me as	Type of self
I am	Actual self
I would really like to be	Ideal self
I used to be	Past self
I should be	Ought self
A new person	Reconstructed self
I hope to become	Expected self
I'm afraid of becoming	Feared self
I could have been	Missed self
Unwanted by one or more others	Rejected self

ACTIVITY 5.2   PRACTICAL

Spend a few minutes going through the different facets of self in the first column (Me as) and see if you can describe yourself in each one. As you are in transition at the moment as a student hoping to become a qualified nurse, you may find it easy. If you do not, you may wish to ask a close friend or family member to help you. Do you agree with the corresponding description of 'types of self'? Remember, these activities are not compulsory so do not feel you have to complete the activity if it makes you feel uncomfortable.

As this activity is based on your own findings, there is no outline answer at the end of the chapter.

Self-disclosure means communicating information about yourself. It may involve information about your values (taking is not as important as giving love); beliefs (I believe the world is square); desires (I would like to fly to the moon and back); behaviour (I eat sweets all day long); or self-qualities or characteristics (I'm always happy). It is a natural part of interpersonal communications and can be verbal or non-verbal. In the former it can be voluntary or as a response to information from another person. In the latter, it can manifest itself in the clothes you wear or the way you speak. However it transpires, it can be best seen in the professional nurse–patient relationship as a developing process in which information is exchanged over a period of time and which changes as the relationship develops from an initial contact to more intimacy and perhaps to eventual deterioration and closure. It depends very much on the nature of the relationship, whether friend, family, parent, child or professional.

Activity 5.3 PRACTICAL

How willing are you to self-disclose? Have a look at the following questions and think about how willing you would be to disclose your answers to a class of fellow students. Score yourself on a 1–4 scale (with 1 as unlikely and 4 as very likely). In the final column, say who you would be most comfortable disclosing this information to.

As this activity is based on your own findings, there is no outline answer at the end of the chapter.

Disclosure	Unlikely 1	Likely 2	Most likely 3	Very likely 4	Preferred person
Some of the happiest moments of your life					
Some of the achievements that you feel particularly proud of					
Aspects of your personality that you don't like					
Your most embarrassing moment					
Your nicknames					
Your greatest fears					

(Adapted from DeVito, 2007)

Activity 5.4 REFLECTIVE

Think for the moment now about patients who are being assessed by you for their health needs. Depending on the nature of their health problems, you may ask them for very intimate information about their hygiene, bowel or urinary functions. You may, if you are undertaking a social history, ask for details of their cohabiting arrangements, family relationships or financial situations. Try to imagine how they feel about divulging this information. Some may anticipate that they will be expected to divulge personal information. For others it may be excruciatingly embarrassing. How can you minimise their discomfort and what is the appropriate amount of self-disclosure you can enter into in this situation?

Some self-disclosure from a nurse in these situations can give an indication of the nurse's understanding of the patient's feelings.

As this activity is based on your own reflection, there is no outline answer at the end of the chapter.

Self-disclosure can be about facts or feelings. When meeting for the first time it is likely that the interaction will be about facts. While you would not be expected to reveal facts about your intimate personal details, you can reveal facts about yourself to equalise the balance, for example how long you have been a nurse or working on the unit. An acknowledgement to the patient that these are personal questions will help create a recognition of the embarrassment factor.

It is accepted in relationships that there is a gradual progression from lower to higher levels of self-disclosure. However, in the professional nurse–patient relationship it has to be accepted that this is not the case. As deeper levels of disclosure are expected from the patient, the nurse's responsibility is to reassure the patient of the confidentiality related to the assessment and establish levels of trust, respect and confidence in the assessment process so that the patient feels comfortable with what will be an imbalance in reciprocity. A major factor is explaining why the information is needed.

Rules of social engagement

In most social situations, we know how to behave because we have learned the **social rules** that govern or guide the interactions. These have evolved from our experiences of family networks and social groups. Examples are the different words we use to initiate an encounter, such as Hello, Hi, How ya doin'?, What's up? and G'day, which all indicate the appropriate response to follow, which would be Hello, Hi, Jus' fine, Not much and Aw right mate.

We have also learned from our regular involvement with activities and events – such as attending lectures, participating in handovers on the unit or having a meal out – the parts we have to play, such as student, staff or friend. This familiarity with social interactions, the expected verbal responses and behaviours gives us a sense of security. We know what to expect, but in new situations, where we might not know the 'rules of engagement' or have an understanding of the shared representations or intersubjective knowledge of what to do, we can feel anxious and isolated. We have to search for clues, observe behaviour patterns or listen to exchanges of information from those already established in the group. This applies to students on their placements for the first time and for patients newly admitted or receiving care for the first time.

RESEARCH SUMMARY

Melia (1984) researched student nurses and found that barriers to socialisation processes were linked to rules. The main thrust of this study was to investigate the occupational socialisation of nursing. Social pressure from staff, and other students, on the wards helped to enforce behaviours that were acceptable to the wards but that did not always put the interests of the patients first. Melia found that, to fit in, students adapted to the new environments by not accepting either the education or service view of acceptable practice. Instead:

Their main concern was to meet the expectations of those with whom they worked, especially those in authority.

(Melia, 1984)

The students thus viewed their training as a series of hurdles to overcome in order to survive.

ACTIVITY 5.5   REFLECTIVE

Do you think your experience as a student is any different now?

How do you think patients feel when they have to reconcile their own world-view of their life and health with that of the hospital, unit or clinic, that is, trying to fit in?

As this activity is based on your own reflection, there is no outline answer at the end of the chapter.

Once the social rules have been learned, people can work and cooperate with a minimum of negotiation. This shared knowledge not only allows us to take for granted social situations, but also makes any kind of adaptation or change to another set of social representations difficult, challenging and at times threatening. Not only do we not know how to behave, because we are so accustomed to behaving in a certain manner, but we associate this with a central perception of ourselves that is also challenged. Our notion of who we are and what role we have to play is compromised and causes, for some people, a profound sense of disequilibrium.

Patients can also experience this disequilibrium when they enter healthcare settings. Understanding their perspective and enabling them to have a clear view of what is expected and the role they have to play can reduce anxiety and make communication more effective.

Making the rules explicit rather than implicit can also help. For example, rules forbidding smoking are explicit. Rules for rewarding or punishing behaviours that are perceived to be bad or do not conform to the shared social rules are not so explicit. This is why patients often do not ask questions – because they are wary of breaking a rule and do not know what the sanctions will be if they do not behave in an expected manner.

Goffman (1972) was a seminal investigator of social rules. An example of how rules determine how we behave was better understood from his studies into the social rules around proximity, personal space and gaze, which are socially and implicitly derived. Humans establish rules concerning the distance they feel comfortable with (see the discussion on 'proxemics' earlier in this chapter, pages 82–3) and the amount of touching that is acceptable between persons. Gaze is crucial in controlling any invasion of this personal space. Looking into someone's eyes implies an intimacy and a closeness, indicating a desire to know someone well. To avoid a 'forced violation of space' or intimacy we look away. No one usually tells you this rule; instead you find it out by observing adults as a child or in social situations in adult life, which is why it is both social and implicit. If you get it wrong you would experience some disfavour or a rebuff, which is the human way to help individuals to learn the rules.

ACTIVITY 5.6 — REFLECTIVE

- What are the social rules of your closest friends?
- When you meet, what are the words you use to signal a friendly greeting and what is the expected response? Has this changed over time?
- Do you use different responses with a different social group?
- How do you signal to each other that you are going to buy the next round of drinks? Or in your group do only the girls buy the drinks?
- How did you learn these codes of behaviour or social rules? Did someone tell you or did you find out by observing others?
- How could it have been made easier to join the group?
- How can you assist patients to understand and become familiar with the social rules of a ward or clinic?

As this activity is based on your own reflection, there is no outline answer at the end of the chapter.

Because of the complexity of these rules, we sometimes cannot avoid breaking a few. To overcome this Goffman suggests minimising the damage by convincing others that we are to be trusted, and that we are competent and worthy. He suggests three tactics.

- Offer an account of why the error happened and give an explanation. This shows that no one is to blame and the error could not be helped – 'I needed to see the other person first because she was just about to go off duty.'

- Offer an apology that accepts part of the blame. This is also an implicit promise that no harm was intended, that you are aware of the rules and that you can be trusted not to transgress again – 'I'm sorry. I don't know why I did that. I knew immediately afterwards that it was wrong.'

- Reconstrue the behaviour as one that was not breaking any rules, but was part of another activity – 'I was only joking.'

There are times when the transgression is too serious and these tactics are insufficient. There is a likelihood that sanctions and damage will follow. Gaining support from colleagues is needed to approach the situation in a professional manner with a plan of action to reduce any harm. Explanations and apologies are required to those who feel injured by the mistakes. Avoiding the mistakes will lead to unresolved guilt on the part of the perpetrator and potential repeated incidents of misunderstanding and mistrust.

The emotional context of communicating

Our emotions are a fundamental part of our personal identity. They can be either pre-programmed (genetic) or learned and they can be demonstrated in many different ways through our actions and interactions. The phrase 'being emotional' is often used to describe someone who is displaying an overtly emotional reaction to a situation by crying, shouting or being upset. Yet we do not always have to display our emotions to know that we are feeling them. Thus, emotions can be either overt or hidden in the depths of our beings. Sometimes we are aware of our emotions and sometimes we are not. This all adds up to fascinating, but complicated, phenomena in the human psyche. Emotions are also connected to the positive or negative values we place on objects, persons and situations. Thus, emotions can colour our perceptions of events and add a layer, or filter, to our experiences, which is intended to help us either cope with the exciting, demanding, unfamiliar and unpleasant or understand the gravity or danger of an experience.

THEORY SUMMARY

The five emotions most often regarded as being fundamental for human beings are as follows.

Happiness	• This includes joy, contentment, having a warm inner glow, feeling like smiling, feeling a sense of well-being, and feeling peace within ourselves. For some, happiness is achieved through pleasure at any cost; for others it is the absence of problems in their lives.
	• Happiness is both transient and enduring.
	• It can differ over cultures.

Fear and anxiety

- Fear is characterised by being afraid of a threat, danger or harm and by being focused on a particular object or experience.
- Anxiety is a generalised, diffused feeling of being threatened without being able to pinpoint the source of the distress.
- In fear, we can point to the cause, in anxiety we cannot.
- Anxiety is more pervasive and tends to last longer.

Anger

- Anger is often precipitated by frustration at not achieving a goal, suffering injustice, or receiving an insult or intentional injury.
- Believing behaviour is unintentional, unavoidable or accidental diminishes anger.
- We are most likely to be angry with people we love than with those we dislike and only slightly towards those we do not know.

Sadness and grief

- Sadness is a mild and relatively brief emotion, whereas grief is a deep and long-lasting period of great sorrow, usually associated with loss.
- Sadness is often caused by making mistakes, being forced to do something against one's judgement, or doing harm to others.
- While it is uncomfortable, sadness has an adaptive quality in that people will try to make redress as a result of sadness.

Disgust

- Disgust is a response to objects or experiences deemed repulsive due to their nature, origin or social history.
- It also has an adaptive function as a motivator to remove ourselves from harm and to reject things that are unsafe.

(Adapted from Dai and Sternberg, 2004)

To the emotions above, you could add surprise, guilt (a private sense of culpability) and shame (public humiliation).

Feelings and emotions allow individuals to experience sensitivity and compassion for another, even though they might not fully understand the situation. In nursing, our emotions are important, as they are an inevitable part of how we respond and react to the persons in our care and to each other. Caring for someone with feeling is also qualitatively different from caring for someone in a distant and dispassionate manner. We utilise the information we receive about how a person is responding, whether it is with happiness, sadness or fear, to judge how we manage the interaction and carry out therapeutic interventions. If a person is very fearful of a procedure, the explanation and management of that person will require specific tuning to that person's needs. If a person is experiencing significant loss or grief over a change in status or disfigurement from a wound, a nurse will adjust the care plan to take into account these feelings, in order to support and enable adjustment to the change in circumstances. A relative or friend who is angry and behaving aggressively because they believe treatment has not been timely or appropriate – often the result of miscommunication or a sense of lack of control – will need sensitive acknowledgement of their fears, worries and frustrations by the nurse and time to assimilate new information.

Balancing emotions

Our aim in life is to have a healthy balance of emotional experiences. This involves letting go of feelings that are damaging or restricting adjustments to new situations and searching for new ways of dealing with situations that provoke emotional responses. This is complicated when a person is unable to express their emotions, which may in turn be a function of not knowing what emotions they are feeling due to confusion, unusual circumstances or changes in the status quo. Alternatively, a person may know what they are feeling but not understand why, or may be experiencing conflicting emotions about the same situation. The nurse's role in these circumstances is to help patients clarify and identify their feelings with the aim of enabling a healthy expression or outlet for the feelings. The best way to do this is to:

- understand the underlying reasons that have provoked the emotional response;
- allow the person to tell their story;
- identify an emotion that is being labelled in the story, for example 'It must be frightening not to understand what is happening to your body right now.'
- ask to help in a non-reactive way, which demonstrates caring by helping to obtain the needed information and validate the fears;
- identify if the person needs a break from the intensity of the situation, for example arrange to come back later to talk over their concerns again.

All these actions are key to developing an understanding and appreciation of the emotional context of a situation from the patient's perspective.

Harmful emotional expression

Emotions can be harmful when they block adjusting to new situations, get out of control or affect another person by reducing their self-esteem. Unresolved feelings can lead to communication misunderstandings in which needs are not perceived to be met. Feelings perceived to be unacceptable can be hidden behind a mask of calm or rationality. Repressed feelings can be expressed with an excessive intensity that is disproportionate to the situation. Consequently, communication and relationships can be distorted by misperceptions created through emotions that are unexpressed, over-expressed or inappropriately expressed. Therefore, the feelings about the content of an interaction have to be balanced with the feelings about what is happening to the self or others in any situation (Hargie, 2006).

CASE STUDY

A nurse has to carry out a procedure on a patient that is going to be uncomfortable, but which is essential to the treatment, for example giving an intramuscular injection. The nurse explains to the patient what is going to happen and why. The patient replies that she hates injections because every injection she has had in the past has been extremely painful and she has never met a nurse who can give an injection without causing bruising. The patient is probably speaking from fear of pain and feels a lack of control. The nurse will feel insecure about his or her skills.

What would you do in this situation?

There is a brief outline answer to this question at the end of the chapter.

Barriers to communication and interpersonal relationships

Before considering the barriers, it is relevant to review the aims of communication and initiating relationships in the healthcare context. From your reading in this book, we hope you will have gathered your own precepts to guide you towards effective interactions; however, here are a few that we hope you have included in your list.

- Establishing a trusting and respectful relationship.
- Transmitting and sharing information.
- Exchanging ideas and understanding perceptions.
- Creating a platform for renewed understanding.
- Enhancing understanding of attitudes, ideas and beliefs.
- Achieving mutually acceptable goals for discourse, interventions and therapy.

An essential ingredient for interactions to be effective is for meanings to be shared and understood. To do this, meanings have to be checked and an awareness created to intercept blocks to communication that can arise from the many differences in individuals, such as authority, power, language, ability and disability, personality, background, gender, health, age, race and socio-economic group.

ACTIVITY 5.7   **PRACTICAL**

What other barriers have you observed in your personal and student experiences that may impede communication?

There is a brief outline answer to this activity at the end of the chapter.

Meaning

It is believed that genuine communication can only be achieved if barriers are identified and worked through. Exploring the meaning, which is an active process created between participants in an interaction between source and receiver, speaker and listener, writer and reader, can help identify some of those barriers. Meaning is not only dependent on messages but also on the interaction between the messages and the thoughts and feelings within those messages. Consequently, meaning is not just 'received'; it is constructed or built up from messages that are received and combined with social and cultural perspectives, for example beliefs, attitudes and values.

It is not just the words that people use; it is the meaning or interpretation that each person gives to the words that construct the meaning. If the understanding of the meaning is shared, there is less likely to be a barrier to communication.

ACTIVITY 5.8   REFLECTIVE

Below are five topical concepts and a potential rating descriptor. Consider each concept and place your own descriptor/word that represents the meaning you have for that concept in the graded column that represents your strength of feeling along a continuum of good to bad. Compare your sense of meanings with a peer.

As this activity is based on your own observations, there is no outline answer at the end of the chapter.

Concept	Good 1	2	3	4	Bad 5
abortion					
terrorism					
schooling					
death penalty					
euthanasia					

An added challenge is that no two persons are likely to derive exactly the same meaning and, because people change their views and ideas about life, it is not always possible to predict accurately another's sense of meaning. Indeed, your own meanings may change from one day to the next depending on your experiences. To refine this process as much as possible, verify the perception you have of another's meanings by asking probing questions, echoing what you perceive to be the other's feelings or thoughts, and seeking elaboration or clarification. In general, practise the communication skills we have discussed in this book. Ultimately, it is wise not to assume that the meaning you attribute to phenomena, actions, situations, behaviours and emotional responses will correspond to another's.

Motivation towards being healthy

One barrier that may impede the nurse–patient relationship is reluctance by the patient to follow health advice. This is a barrier associated with a person's beliefs about the cause of their illness or their health and well-being. Advising patients to follow treatment regimes or adopt different lifestyle choices to maintain or improve their health requires a detailed understanding of how health beliefs are constructed. It requires a concentrated form of communication that builds upon the strategies already presented, but that may be content-specific in contrast to the free-flowing therapeutic style. This is because the nurse is deliberately including information for the patient to hear and understand, and which has consequences for the future health of the patient. There is also a clearer expectation of the outcome, which is that the patient will follow a medication regime, or undertake specific daily activities that may require learning a different or new set of skills.

There are several models in the literature that guide this process. Role performance models evaluate functioning and successful outcomes as benchmarks of achievement in adopting new health behaviours. Adaptive models consider self-care approaches to alteration in behaviours. Self-fulfilment has also been incorporated into these models, borrowed from Maslow's hierarchy of needs and the **eudaemonistic** model proposed by Smith (1987).

Pender et al. (2006) have devised a model that is more comprehensive and value based towards positive well-being and health. It borrows from the health belief model and incorporates motivational factors. The aim of the model is to explore how an individual perceives their health status through cognitive-perceptual factors, such as self-efficacy, control over health, and benefits and barriers to health. It also takes into account modifying factors, such as immunisations, family histories, individual personality and characteristics, situational factors and the influences of others.

ACTIVITY 5.9   PRACTICAL

Go to the Pender websites (URLs are at the end of this chapter) and read the propositions underpinning Pender's health promotion model. Identify a barrier you, a friend or relative may have towards adopting health advice. If possible, interview that friend or relative, or undertake a self-assessment of the factors that are influencing taking health advice.

How would you use the information you have gathered in this exercise in your future practice?

As this activity is based on your own observations, there is no outline answer at the end of the chapter.

Conflict

It may be difficult to accept, but it is widely agreed by many writers that there are times in every relationship when those involved will agree to differ, and the healthcare context is no exception. Misunderstandings arise when conflict is experienced and it is assumed that there is something wrong with the situation or that the relationship is in jeopardy or damaged. A difference of opinion is not a conflict; it is where two sets of creative thought or ideas differ. The situation that becomes misunderstood or develops into an aggressive outburst is one where the misunderstandings have expanded to include personal egos, lack of trust and emotional perceptions that distort the relativity of the situation. The role of the nurse in situations of conflict is to be aware of the dynamics and the skills required for resolution.

Conflict can serve as an alarm to indicate that a relationship needs closer attention. It sometimes offers an opportunity to clarify differences of opinion and in a therapeutic relationship may be necessary to work towards achieving a different set of behaviours or responses from the patient. The disadvantages of conflict are increasing negativity, hurting others and depleting energy that is needed for other emotional tasks. The positive effects are that it can lead to a closer examination of issues that are rearing up in a relationship or group. Examining the problems and finding solutions to the conflict can be a way to mend bridges and strengthen relationships. Nonetheless, experiencing conflict can be disquieting and uncomfortable, giving rise to feelings that can be challenging or in opposition to closely held beliefs or values.

The first step in conflict resolution is to analyse the situation. Arnold and Boggs (2007) state that the things to consider are:

- previous experiences with conflict situations;
- the degree to which the conflict is acceptable;
- the intensity of the feeling it arouses;
- the physical, cognitive and emotional health or stamina of the persons involved;
- the subjective interpretation of the event or conflict;
- the consequences.

Conflict can become manageable when the causes, sources and issues underpinning the conflict are clearly articulated by the parties involved. This needs time and the use of non-judgemental listening skills to collect the stories. By drawing out hidden feelings or repressed ideas that otherwise may not have been known, barriers to communication can be identified and resolved.

One of the commonest responses to conflict is to become angry. As mentioned above, anger is one of our fundamental emotions and it originates in a part of the brain called the amygdala, which is responsible for thought and judgements. The anger response is intended to identify threats and prepare our bodies for attack. This is a rapid response that is very necessary in life-threatening situations; however, it does not always give us time to think about appropriate responses or the consequences of our actions.

THEORY SUMMARY

The human response to conflict is defensive and this can be aggressive; however, there are three forms of aggressive behaviour: aggressive, passive or passive-aggressive. The aggressive response is to deflect the attack through personal attack or blaming, generating feelings in the other person of anger and resentment. The passive response is self-preservation by not engaging or by wishing to resolve the conflict. This generates feelings of frustration and loss of respect. The passive-aggressive response is where, on the surface, a person appears to be agreeing to plans and arrangements that are made, but in reality is not engaging with the activities designed to solve the problems. There can be verbal agreement at the same time as sabotaging or discrediting activities undertaken by the passive-aggressor, which leads to confusion and mistrust.

ACTIVITY 5.10   PRACTICAL

With a group of peers, identify the sources of conflict that you have witnessed in the clinical areas you have experienced so far. Separate out those situations that involved staff to staff, staff to patients and vice versa, and patient to patient. Analyse these situations to identify common features of the causes of conflict.

What examples have you witnessed of good conflict management? Compare these with poorly managed examples.

As this activity is based on your own observations, there is no outline answer at the end of the chapter.

The second step in conflict resolution is to identify the potential solutions to the problems or issues that are causing the conflict. Key elements for any professional involved in a conflict situation are to remember that the rights of the individuals involved are to be respected and to behave in an assertive manner. Assertiveness needs to be learned and the websites listed at the end of the chapter will provide you with some resources to work through. If you are going to set up a meeting to resolve conflict, Arnold and Boggs (2007) suggest that you will need to consider the following.

- Prepare for the encounter – be clear about the purpose, what the major points to discuss are going to be and whether the information you have is complete and can be shared. Give careful consideration to the language used and the choice of words so that messages are clear and unambiguous.

- Organise your information and consult with another to validate your approach, preferably someone who is objective. Rehearse.

- Manage your own anxiety – use breathing and relaxation techniques to calm you. Think of a mantra to reinforce your commitment to your rights.
- Time the encounter – judge when parties will be receptive, allow time for discussion and expressions of choice and be prepared to listen.
- Take one issue at a time and focus on the present – break the problem down into small units or steps and allow time for clarification. If one small area can be resolved, this can lead to further resolutions.
- Request a change in behaviour or response – assess the level of readiness and take into consideration maturity, culture, values and life factors.
- Evaluate the conflict resolution – it may take more time; small goals can be achieved first. Aim for a climate of openness and future communication.

Taking steps to solve problems and reduce conflict requires skilled handling and can be achieved through observation and practice in role play.

ACTIVITY 5.11   PRACTICAL

Take one of the incidents you have witnessed and ask a peer to role play the incident and go through the stages outlined above. Take a turn each at the two different sides of the conflict to experience what it feels like and to practise the dialogue.

As this activity is based on your own observations, there is no outline answer at the end of the chapter.

CHAPTER SUMMARY

In this chapter we have explored relationship boundaries between professional relationships and friendships/kinships. We have also looked at relevant research and the implications of intimacy and proximity. Emotions, and how they need to be balanced to achieve effective communication outcomes, have been discussed and you should now understand the construction of meaning and how this underpins communication messages. We have stressed the importance of interpreting meanings to clarify understanding and perceptions of events, and you should have learned how motivation factors can affect health messages, and how to identify the benefits and barriers to achieving health-promoting communications. We have also explained how conflicts can arise and how they should be handled in healthcare settings

Activities: brief outline answers

Case study (pages 79–80)

There is potential for this situation to become a power study and cause loss of self-esteem for the nurse. The key is to acknowledge the patient's underlying sense of fear and apprehension. Is it due to fear of pain or lack of confidence in the staff, or uncertainty about why this treatment is necessary? By clarifying the reasons for the emotions, the nurse can help to put the patient at ease. This will also establish a relationship that is more than just carrying out a procedure and one that can be productive in the future.

Activity 5.7 (page 92)

Barriers to communication that you may have observed include:

- organisational structures;
- pressure of limited available time;
- involvement of other people;
- the physical environment;
- interruptions;
- fear, anxiety, embarrassment or lack of self-confidence;
- lack of information.

KNOWLEDGE REVIEW

Having completed the chapter, how would you now rate your knowledge of the following topics?

	Good	Adequate	Poor
1. The relevance of the professional relationship in CIPS.			
2. How emotions can impact communication.			
3. The construction and interpretation of meaning in interpersonal interactions.			
4. How conflicts can be resolved.			

Where you're not confident in your knowledge of a topic, what will you do next?

Further reading

Arnold, E and Boggs, KU (2007) *Interpersonal Relationships: Professional communication skills for nurses*, 5th edition. Philadelphia, PA: WB.Saunders.

Useful websites

www.businessballs.com/self-confidence-assertiveness.htm A website with information on assertiveness training.

www.mentalhelp.net/poc/center_index.php?id=116&cn=116 A site about anger management – has many resources on explaining the physiology and psychology of anger as well as techniques for managing angry outbursts.

www.nursing.umich.edu/faculty/pender/chart.gif This website has information about Pender's health promotion model.

www.nursing.umich.edu/faculty/pender/HPM.pdf Another site about Pender's health promotion model, including assumptions and theoretical propositions.

6. The learning and educational context

CHAPTER AIMS

After reading this chapter, you will be able to:

- describe how to integrate theory and practice;
- understand the importance of learning from experience, so that learning can be based on reality;
- know what is expected at the different levels of learning;
- manage reflection in portfolios for assessment;
- identify activities to enhance communication in learning and teaching situations;
- commit yourself to lifelong learning.

Introduction

You will have many learning goals in your time as a student and this chapter will guide you in achieving these through enhanced communication and interpersonal skills (CIPS). So far in this book we have been focusing on CIPS for your role as a professional. In this chapter we will be focusing on how CIPS can support you and your individual learning pathway – now and throughout your career. The way we will do this is to look at a spectrum of your role as learner through to educator and eventually your own continuing learning needs as a lifelong learner (see Figure 6.1).

This chapter will examine each of these three stages in the spectrum, beginning with a discussion on you as a student and learner. We will explore some of the issues related to the integration of theory and practice. This leads us to discuss how learning should be realistic and relevant to your practice and learning needs. One way to achieve this is through experiential learning techniques, which we will explore through a model. Learning through experience is regarded as learning by doing, rather than by listening to others or reading. This form of learning involves active, rather than passive, learning through interactions, self-awareness, expression, flexibility and reciprocity, and with relevance or meaning. All these characteristics are present in CIPS as they are very much related to how you behave in interpersonal situations. Consequently, learning through experience, which refers to deliberately planned learning experiences, and learning from experience, which refers to past experiences to gain new insights, are two highly relevant learning approaches in CIPS.

Following this, a framework for levels of academic qualifications is presented with a discussion on how this links to practice. The skills gained from examining this framework will enable you to operate more effectively within complex care

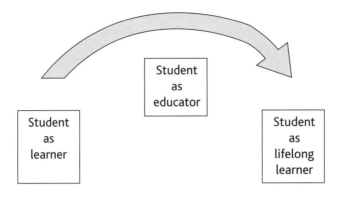

Figure 6.1: Spectrum of learner, educator and lifelong learner.

environments for decision making, and will facilitate problem solving, critical thinking and reflective capacities. We have drawn links to the assessment of practice requirements to enable you to have a clearer idea of how to gain proficiency in skills. We have also included sections on reflective writing, learning styles and the characteristics of a skilled performance, which will help you complete your practice learning assessments and put CIPS into practice.

There are many different contexts in which students can act as educators among colleagues and with patients, in order to give instruction or guidance on health promotion or health education perspectives. Guidelines for improving communication in these settings are provided, along with a description of the professional standards required in these circumstances.

The final section of the chapter looks to the future and considers the role of a student in formulating a frame of mind to include lifelong learning. We look at the importance of skills from a health policy perspective and consider the extended scope of practice through career trajectories and forward thinking.

Student as learner

Integration of theory and practice

One of the constant dilemmas for nursing students during their studies is striving to integrate the theories learned in the classroom with the practice of nursing performed in clinical, real-world situations. This is no easier with CIPS, which can seem so obvious and yet, as this book demonstrates, are not just simple skill sets to be learned in a rote fashion. We all have CIPS abilities and what has to be achieved during studies is enhancing, improving and making more effective these skills in healthcare settings. We have already explored some theories in this book and have attempted to use practical exercises to demonstrate how the theory can be applied. Judging how meaningful these are and how they can be applied to good effect helps with the integration of theory with practice. But it may not be enough.

The NMC *Standards of Proficiency* (2004a) argue that practice, integrated with theory, needs to be evidence-based, thus safe. In Chapter 2, we explored the importance of integrating theory with practice and the relationship to research that provides the evidence for safe practice. As with any practice-based skill, practice makes perfect and this applies equally to CIPS. Practising using the skills by working with models in an environment that is safe, exactly in the same way that you might practise inserting a naso-gastric tube, is as essential as rehearsing practical skills. The difference may be the self-consciousness or self-awareness you may have as you say words that are unfamiliar or use phrases that, at first, sound false and stilted. The conditions you need in order to practise are therefore important.

ACTIVITY **6.1**   REFLECTIVE

What are the ideal conditions that you need in order to practise a new communication or interpersonal skill?

Do you need to be alone and in front of a mirror? With a close friend, or in a group? Each of these situations can pose different levels of complexity in communication, how you use your interpersonal skills and the feedback you will get on the effectiveness of your skills.

As this activity is based on your own reflection, there is no outline answer at the end of the chapter.

Disconcertingly, there is continuing evidence that final-year nursing students and immediately post-qualifying nurses have difficulty sustaining the values and ideals they gained during their training (Maben et al., 2006, 2007; Jasper, 1996). Maben et al. (2006) found that, while nurses had gained a strong set of values during their programmes of study, there were professional and organisational factors that prevented them from taking their ideas into practice. The study felt that this had serious consequences for the integration of theory with practice, as the need to obey covert rules, lack of support and poor role models inhibited newly qualified nurses in carrying out their ideas of evidenced-based practice and appropriate standards of care. There were additional demands, such as time pressures, constraints on roles – that is, boundaries and opportunities – shortages of staff and work overload. By practising and applying the ideas, concepts and theories (the summaries of how these concepts are organised) during and beyond your course, you will be working towards closing the theory–practice gap.

Learning for reality

Eve Bendall (1976) was one of the first nurse researchers to study the theory–practice gap. In her seminal work on how students learn clinical skills, which she called learning for reality, she found that, by observing students in practice and comparing this with what they wrote, they described one thing in writing and then did something completely different in practice. The assumption was that a written description by a student nurse would be sufficient evidence to judge that the nurse was competent to carry out care for specific patient conditions. Her study found the assumption to be false and was pivotal in formulating the practise-based curriculum that nurses experience today.

Today's nurses are deemed to be more patient-focused and more effective with social interaction. This is credited to the inclusion of theoretical concepts drawn from the social sciences into nursing care. These are integrated into theoretical models of nursing specifically designed to guide care, yet nursing remains a practice-based profession requiring the demonstration of skills proficiencies. Over time, nursing skills have expanded from purely physical activities with, for example, visual, auditory, verbal, tactile, kinaesthetic and organisational factors, to include those underpinned by the social sciences, including, for example, the psychological, social, interactive, interpretive and conceptual factors we are exploring in this book (Bendall, 2006).

To enable nurses to learn practical skills, there are different viewpoints on how this can best be achieved. One view is that principles should be taught early in the course, so that they can then be taken to the practice settings and applied and practised in different situations until competency is reached. In this approach, evidence-based care is taken to the practice area and carried out in vivo – in the living and real environment. The tasks are supervised by a qualified mentor and then assessed.

Another view is for students to observe care being delivered and for the elements of nursing care in any one situation to be identified by the students. So, for example, in a practice setting the nurse carries out different actions with and for the patients. The task of the student is to make note of these activities and assemble these into a whole picture of care that is required for that particular setting. Once assembled, the student follows up the tasks to discover if there is evidence underpinning the activities, discriminates between the essential or unessential elements and determines if there are sequences or levels of ordering in the elements to enable them to apply the activities when they are required to do so without supervision. This is a more complex method, but is more detailed, and requires mentors to establish whether or not students have identified the relevant parts of the whole, their relative significance and appropriateness in the situation.

Each of these approaches has advantages. The first is that students are prepared with ideas and strategies before they enter the practice setting. Many students find this comforting, as they do not wish to be seen as incompetent when they first go into practice. It also enables students to feel confident about a situation that has the potential to undermine their confidence. The second is based on the **Gestalt** idea that all experiences are based on the sum of the individual parts and that, by examining the parts, a whole can be assembled with better understanding of how the parts interact. The term 'gestalt' is derived from the German term meaning 'pattern' or 'configuration' and this enables learning. The patterns are thought to stand out from the background against which they are seen, giving rise to the concepts of figure and ground in perceiving phenomena.

Experiential learning

A third approach to practice learning is through experiential learning. This is where individuals go through a process of experiencing, reflecting, thinking and acting. Kolb and Fry (1975) proposed this theory, which claims that experiencing a phenomenon leads to observations and reflections. They believed that these activities form a cycle of activities that make up a four-stage learning cycle. Feeling in this context does not describe an emotional experience, although that may contribute to the experience. Feeling is intended to mean a perceived physical or mental sensation. It could also relate to a particular impression, appearance, effect or atmosphere sensed from something, such as a feeling of abandonment about a building. We cannot also rule out that feeling can relate to an instinctive awareness or presentiment of something, such as a prediction that someone will be disappointed with some news. A simple model of these activities is represented in Figure 6.2.

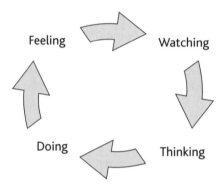

Figure 6.2: A simplistic model of Kolb and Fry's experiential learning theory.

Kolb and Fry originally based this model on their work with groups. The model has been further adapted to include the processes of reviewing data and information that will happen during thinking about the experience. The next stage is to puzzle out or give some meaning to the experience. This is then added to the ideas that will influence any further experiences or responses to situations (see Figure 6.3). The main premise is that we all have an intrinsic tendency to draw upon our experiences of the world we live in. This helps us to improve our knowledge of what happens to us, and to formulate our opinions and extend our range of skills and knowledge.

We are constantly taking in information through our senses and digesting this information as we experience events, which means that we are never completely in static situations. Even those folk who give the appearance of 'switching off' are still receiving some information, although they wish to give the impression that they are not dealing with it for one reason or another, such as tiredness, dislike of a situation or, in the case of illness, pain and discomfort. They are deliberately turning off that engagement switch or, more likely, tuning down.

Using experience to guide our actions and beliefs does, however, present its challenges. If we only gauge our current reactions based on previous experiences,

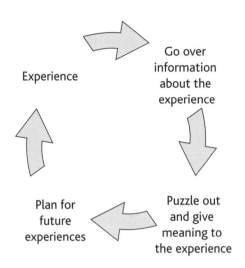

Figure 6.3: Experiential learning cycle.

we are, in fact, limited only to those previous experiences. While our experiences may stand us in good stead in most situations, they may also not always provide us with sufficient solutions to the problems we have to solve. We cannot have experienced every phenomenon in the world in preparation for the next experience, whatever that may be. Thus, our wisdom is limited by our past experiences.

Our decisions to base our actions on previous experiences may also be founded on assumptions, whether 'true' or 'false', and either our conscious or unconscious assimilation of ideas. It is the stage of the cycle where we ascribe meaning to events and experiences. By interpreting the experiences, and in an attempt to understand why something is happening, we use different strategies to give an event meaning. Meaning can be divined from the symbolism of an event, such as a memorial service, which means sadness; here, the concrete symbolises the abstract. Or it can be drawn from the notion of what the significance or magnitude of an event represents to someone. Some experiences will therefore have more significance to some than others. Meaning can also be constructed from a moral or psychological sense that relates to a sense of purpose or reason.

We rely on our previous experiences to guide our responses but do not necessarily learn from, or adjust, our responses to improve how we react in situations. Most of the time we store our memories of experiences in 'cold storage' or classify them as 'unfinished business' to be returned to when we have enough psychological energy. This explanation can help us understand why some people never learn from experience, because they never return to the cold storage of their memories. To enable us to learn from those experiences we need to combine 'here and now' learning and reflection (see Siviter and Stevens (2004) for practical guidance on surviving as student nurse).

This is the essence of experiential learning. It is not just learning to do something differently next time, but is more about actively engaging in an analysis and reflection on what has been learned, how it compares with previous learning and how this accumulative store of learning can be built upon further to improve skills and knowledge. This is so relevant when learning about CIPS. You will have already stored up many experiences of your own and will have also refined some of your interpersonal skills as a result of those experiences.

ACTIVITY 6.2   REFLECTIVE

Take a moment to think about a communication misunderstanding that you have experienced. Now take a moment to think about what you learned from that experience. What was your interpretation of it? How would you improve your communication of information in that experience the next time you face a similar situation?

As this activity is based on your own reflection, there is no outline answer at the end of the chapter.

In nursing, students are given time to learn in practice under the guidance of mentors or experienced healthcare practitioners. In the same way that you learn to carry out a physical procedure, it is important first to observe communication and interpersonal interactions. You can then practise under supervision and be prepared to undertake communication of information on your own. At each stage of the process, you will continue to learn and you will need to create opportunities to review what you are learning, clarify what you have learned from past experiences and think about future experiences to extend your skills. So that you can also gain optimally from these experiences, it is important to know when you are learning by experience as distinct from learning from experience.

Learning by experience is more or less an unconscious process. It is a realisation after the experience that we have learned something significant. These experiences are gained through the reality of professional life, varying and unpredictable demands and changing circumstances. An example of this is that we can often be so preoccupied with getting something right that, when we forget to try and we get it right, there is a sudden integration of knowledge and surprise that the skill can be mastered after all.

To draw optimally from these experiences, you need to hone your skills of attention to both external events and what you are experiencing internally. Internal processes include noticing your thoughts, intuitions, emotions, bodily sensations, intentions for yourself and others, needs, what you are doing, how you are doing it and how all this relates together (see Figure 6.4).

There is a balance to be struck between being immersed in an experience and totally absorbed by it, and being a witness. So that you can learn from the experience, ask yourself the following questions.

Similar situations
- Expectations
- The act of trying to remember and memorising
- Brainstorming
- Evaluating

Creative new ideas
- Imaginations
- Hunches and guesses
- Images
- Memories of past meetings

Problem solving
- Rehearsing
- Visualising
- Forecasting
- Understanding

Figure 6.4:
Examples of thoughts
and intuitions.

- What am I thinking/feeling/noticing now that describes this situation?
- Am I experiencing any tensions in my body?
- What am I imagining and assuming or presuming?

To help you become more aware, begin to verbalise your thoughts and feelings about experiences to fellow students or mentors.

Learning from experience is a more deliberate and conscious experience. The intention is not just to experience the 'here and now', but to devise future actions based on the reflection and evaluation of events.

Using the experiential learning cycle (look back to Figure 6.3 on page 105) requires time for thinking and reflection. Some of this goes on informally in social groups or at the end of a shift with groups of peers. The more aware we become of our feelings and intuitions about experiences and the comparison of these reflections of both inner and outer experiences, the more objective our memories of the experiences will be. By practising using the experiential cycle, students can begin to work through the stages without checking where they are at each stage. Thus, the process of reflection becomes integrated as an evaluative process for refining skills. This will serve to enhance the reflections and learning through experience to greater effect.

Levels of learning

Many students ask lecturers what is wanted from them as they progress from one level of learning to another. One reason for this is that students want to see how they are progressing during their studies and how they are improving or, as we have said above, enhancing their skills and knowledge. A starting point is to decide what is meant by levels in relation to learning in higher education (HE).

Diplomas, degrees and postgraduate courses have the levels determined by the Higher Education Funding Council (HEFC) of the UK, which utilises standards set by the Quality Assurance Agency (QAA) in a framework for academic achievement (the Qualification Framework in Higher Education). The QAA has produced a booklet for students explaining the qualifications framework (see 'Useful websites' at the end of this chapter) and has identified five levels, three of which are undergraduate and two postgraduate, as shown in the box below.

Table 6.1: Qualifications framework

Certificate	C Level	Certificates of Education.
Intermediate	I Level	Foundation degrees, ordinary Bachelor's degrees, Diplomas of Higher Education, and other Higher Diplomas.
Degree	D level	Bachelor's degrees with honours, Graduate Certificates and Graduate Diplomas.
Masters	M level	Master's degrees, Postgraduate Certificates and Postgraduate Diplomas.
Doctoral	D level	Doctorates.

Each level has a descriptor outlining what is expected and demonstrates the nature of change at each level. The descriptors are further subdivided into two parts. In the first part are the outcomes against which the awards will be judged and granted. The second part describes the wider, more general, abilities a student should be able to achieve after following such a programme and is intended to inform employers.

ACTIVITY 6.3   PRACTICAL

Go to the QAA website (www.qaa.ac.uk/academicinfrastructure/FHEQ/EWNI/ default.asp#annex1), explore for yourself the descriptors and examine whether or not you are achieving these for yourself.

Think about what you need to do to extend your ability to achieve the levels for your intended level of study. You may find that these general descriptors are insufficient to describe what and how you are learning, because they are brief or because they do not include practice descriptors.

As this activity is based on your own findings, there is no outline answer at the end of the chapter.

In nursing we have the additional descriptors, or standards of proficiency, that the NMC requires to be completed before professional registration as a nurse can be assured. They are appropriately heavily slanted towards practice, so they, too, have a limitation if they are seen to be external to or exclude the theory work we are also undertaking in our courses.

To overcome this, a model used by the Southern England Consortium for Credit Accumulation and Transfer (known as SEEC) has been favoured by many institutions as it includes a reference to practical skills in conjunction with knowledge gained through a progressive hierarchy. The levels were devised as a response to the changing face of HE, where academic levels could no longer always be described in close relation to years of study. For example, an undergraduate programme would always be three years when, with the success of the Open University providing flexible learning opportunities, a student could take up to six years to complete a degree. Also, courses were changing to include elements or modules within courses that required a framework to clarify the level and the extent of academic effort required to complete these elements. A definition of an academic level in this context has therefore been given as:

> *An indicator of relative demand, complexity, depth of study and learner autonomy.*
>
> (Gosling and Moon, 2001, p8)

Before moving on to examine the **level descriptors** provided by the SEEC, we can think about the general expectations that can be used to map or guide the level at which you are functioning with your CIPS in the following activity.

Activity 6.4   Practical

Think of a recent interaction you have had with a patient who asked you to help solve a problem or correct a misunderstanding concerning their treatment or illness. Write down a short account of the episode. It does not have to be a situation that you regard as being particularly satisfactory or, conversely, needing improvement; just be spontaneous here.

Then analyse the situation using the following steps and questions.

1. How would you rate the *complexity of knowledge and understanding* you need to undertake this interaction from 1 to 5 (5 being highly complex and involving detailed knowledge). Was it an everyday situation or were you thinking on your feet because you had not encountered this situation before? Did you have to draw on some knowledge gleaned from one of your sessions at the university or some nugget of information that your mentor had recently shared with you? Did something you had read in a nursing journal or textbook come to mind? Were you aware of any ethical issues underpinning or influencing this situation?

2. How would you rate your *standard of cognitive skills*? Were you able to *analyse* and break down the elements of the situation into segments that enabled you to understand the situation better? Did it help you when you put back the parts of the interaction to see a different aspect to the relationship you have with the patient, or identify influences and ideas? This would be *synthesising* information. To what extent did you make a judgement on the value, importance, extent or condition of the situation and interaction between you and the patient? This would constitute your *evaluation* of the situation.

   How did steps 1 and 2 affect your response and behaviour towards the patient? This would be the result of your thinking or cognitive processes and application of your knowledge.

3. The third step is to assess your ability to use *generic* or *transferable skills*. These are life skills that you acquire through extending your learning opportunities. You should ask yourself if you have drawn on any of the experiences you have had from working with your fellow students or teams in your practice experience (i.e. *group working*). Have you learned to react differently, or use new or different phrases to express yourself, in order to help you be more clearly understood by patients and colleagues? Are you willing to put effort into your learning or do you expect it all to be easy and not to require any additional work (*ethos towards learning*)? Did you turn to any learning resources, books, articles or the internet to help you understand this situation more fully, and how effective did you think you were in finding, synthesising and utilising the resources (*use of learning resources and management of information*)? Do you rely on others to find things out or do you actively go and independently seek out information for your studies to improve your knowledge (*autonomy*)? How do you know if your communication style was appropriate and effective? When you report back to

another member of the team, how clear were you in recounting the situation (*communication*)? Were there potentially different solutions to choose from in this situation and do you think you applied the correct solution to the situation you recounted (*problem solving*)? How would you rate your ability to choose the most appropriate method, treatment, or answer to correct a problem (*self-evaluation*)?

4. The fourth step is to identify if you were acting with the appropriate level of *responsibility* in this situation? Who was responsible? A qualified nurse or medical practitioner? Was it the patient's responsibility or that of the patient's family? Did the organisation have a role to play in this situation? Did you, or who did, have the authority to make independent decisions this situation?

5. Was it appropriate that you responded to the patient or should you have consulted with a qualified nurse? To what *level of independence* are you able to apply your learning?

6. How much *guidance* do you require in these situations? It is quite acceptable to say that you still require guidance because you are still a student; however, you should be thinking about what activities you can undertake confidently and competently and plan to work independently on some activities now or at a point in the future for more complex situations.

As this activity is based on your own observations, there is no outline answer at the end of the chapter.

All the phrases and words highlighted in italic in the above activity are key words in the descriptors for estimating levels of learning. If you ask yourself these questions each time you undertake an assessment or want to improve your CIPS, you will be extending your own levels of learning (see the guidance on study skills in Taylor (2003)).

In Appendix 1 of the document *How to Use Level Descriptors* by Jenny Moon (2002), you will find detailed information of what is expected at every level, including descriptors for practical skills. As a general rule, you should be achieving level 1 at the end of your Common Foundation year. If you are following a diploma course, you should be demonstrating level 2 by the end of your course and, if you are following a degree course, you should be working towards demonstrating level 3 by the end of your course.

Assessment of practice in portfolios

Bearing in mind that you need to demonstrate a wide range of thinking skills alongside your development of practice skills, there remains the thorny issue of how both theory (which is an intellectual activity related to your thinking skills) and practice can be captured in one place to demonstrate the achievement of competence. One method is by using portfolios of evidence. Since the early 1990s, portfolios were used to capture evidence of nursing students' learning in practice. Over the years, these have been consistently developed and improved from initially being bulky repositories for sheaves of paper to slimmer versions providing a succinct method for collating evidence. They have now become an integral part of the majority of nursing education programmes (see Maslin-Prothero (2005) for further guidance).

Reflective writing

It is generally agreed that **reflective writing** is considered the key to assessment by portfolio. This is because it provides evidence of the development of skills and can demonstrate increasing clinical competence over a period of time. We would expect to see development over time as you cannot expect to be competent straightaway. Smith (1997) found some evidence that reflection assisted the integration of practice experience with academic knowledge. Development over time was also another feature of this study. However, in a study by Smith and Jack (2005) students were asked if reflection was a meaningful activity and no consensus of opinion was reached. The authors did find that the students' learning style was highly pertinent to their perception of the usefulness of reflection (see Rolfe et al. (2001) for further guidance on reflection).

Learning styles

There are several theories on learning styles and these have been reviewed by Coffield et al. (2004). The majority focus around three or four main attributes. Two of the most widely used are the learning style inventories of Kolb (2000) (whose experiential learning theory we examined earlier in this chapter) and of Honey and Mumford (1992). Both of these versions can easily be found on the internet for you to test out yourself (see 'Useful websites' at the end of the chapter). Essentially, Kolb's inventory suggests that we each have a preference for one of four styles: concrete experience (feeling), reflective observation (watching), abstract conceptualisation (thinking) and active experimentation (doing). These are clustered into two continuums with conflicting axes: feeling and thinking vs. watching and doing. He believes that we choose to learn by grasping at an experience to transform it into something that is meaningful and useful. Our learning styles are therefore a product of these two decisions: either preferring to watch and do, or thinking and feeling.

Honey and Mumford, however, believe there are also four dimensions to learning styles. They describe these as characteristics and divide people into activists, who learn by doing, reflectors, who stand back and observe first, theorists, who prefer to adapt and integrate experiences into a conceptual whole or framework, and pragmatists, who, while on the look out for new ideas, will only adopt ideas if they have a practical benefit. There are some similarities between the two approaches to learning styles, but you may want to ponder over which is your preferred style, as the research suggests that those students who could relate to the tasks through meaningful reflection were best able to utilise the experience of portfolio learning and the impact that reflection could have on their learning. Therefore, identifying which is your preferred learning style will help you recognise the effort you will require in another style on the axis of the dimensions to become more reflective if, for example, you are primarily a pragmatist or 'doing' learner. Your approach to reflection as a learning strategy will improve and you will have a more positive outlook towards this form of learning. This is borne out by a study of pre-clinical medical students undertaken by Rees and Sheard (2004), who found that students who were more positive about reflective portfolios were more likely to rate their reflection skills as good, achieve higher marks for their portfolios and have more confidence in building future portfolios.

RESEARCH SUMMARY

If you are a person who finds reflection difficult and who has a tendency to pragmatism and learning only for reality, you may want to consider the research of Teekman (2000) on exploring reflection in nursing practice using a sense-making approach. He searched for sense-making activities in a group of qualified nurses to examine how they made sense of situations as well as their thought processes. He found that reflective thinking was apparent in moments of doubt and perplexity, categorising perceptions, framing and self-questioning to gain sense and understanding of what was happening in situations. You may be using reflective thinking without realising if you have ever had a mental tussle over what to do in a difficult situation. You now need to use those same thinking activities and apply them to all situations. This will help you delve deeper into your levels of learning and improve your analytical abilities. In the sense-making theory utilised in Teekman's research, situations are identified as the inexplicable inconsistencies of human experience that are influenced by culture, social organisation and individual perception. There is then a gap where the individual is stopped in their tracks (that is, in a state of discontinuity), where routine thinking is no longer applicable and where new constructions or solutions are required in order to create a personal sense of the situation. 'Uses' is the last stage of the activity, where the individual puts the new thinking into practical use.

Skilled performance

While you may now realise that experiential learning, reflective writing and your preferred learning style may influence how you achieve your learning goals in the assessment of your practice, you will want to know what makes a skilled performance stand out when practice is being assessed. Some essential characteristics are outlined below.

Accuracy	Skill executed with precision.
Speed	Movements are swift and confident.
Efficiency	Movements are economical, with the ability to draw upon additional movement when required.

Timing	Accurate timing and correct sequential order.
Consistency	Results are consistent, and repeated successfully on different occasions.
Anticipation	Can anticipate events very quickly and respond accordingly.
Adaptability	Can adapt the skill to current circumstances.
Perception	Can obtain maximum information from a minimum of cues.

As mentioned before, any skill has to be practised before it is learned. The more you practise your communication skills with colleagues and friends, and think about the different situations that require different responses, the more it will help you refine your skills and improve your confidence. You are also advised to hone your observational skills and make notes of situations in, for example, the classroom, waiting rooms, clinics and in practice,. Evaluate these interactions and conjure up scenarios where you would improve your skills. By developing the skills of observation and analysis, inviting feedback and considering the context in which nursing practice takes place, your critical reflection skills will also develop and you will avoid any negatively framed, overly introspective analysis.

Student as educator

You may only regard yourself as a student who is there to learn rather than teach. But we would propose that there will be opportunities when you will find yourself giving an explanation, directions, instructions or a presentation, or untangling a misunderstanding, and you will be – in effect – teaching another person some aspect of healthcare (see Arnold and Boggs (2004) for detailed help on teaching health promotion and health education). This could be teaching a fellow student either in the practice setting or in the classroom, a patient concerning their health or disease, or even qualified staff if you are presenting a project you have undertaken as part of your studies. There are many self-help texts around to guide you with teaching skills, which is why in this chapter we will be concentrating on how you can communicate clearly, using interpersonal skills effectively to transmit information when you act as an educator (see Quinn and Hughes, 2007).

Health communication skills

Because there are so many factors affecting healthcare communications, it is difficult to refine the competencies into a 'laundry list', yet interprofessional communication can improve the chances of communicating effectively. Seven top health communication skills have been organised from different research studies and are outlined briefly here.

1 Giving accurate and sufficient feedback

Feedback is a message sent back to the message sender to give reassurance that the message has been received and understood. For example, it is reassuring for a patient to receive feedback that they have been understood or for you to receive reassurance from the patient that they have understood you. Do not be afraid to give positive feedback to encourage performance and to gain clarity in a situation. If you are uncertain whether something has been clearly understood, ask for confirmation or ask if any further explanation is required. Alternatively, if you see an inaccuracy in performance and you are certain that there is another way in which a procedure can be carried out, and more effectively, you need to say so in a manner that is without prejudice or malice.

ACTIVITY 6.5   PRACTICAL

You may want to practise giving feedback to your close friends and ask them how it felt. Similarly, let them practise on you, so that you can experience what it is like and discover the most appropriate and acceptable phrases to use in these situations.

As this activity is based on your own observations, there is no outline answer at the end of the chapter.

Non-verbal feedback is equally important, as it registers reactions to what has been said, for example facial expressions such as surprise, boredom or hostility. Behaviours such as leaving the room or remaining silent are also non-verbal indicators of feedback!

ACTIVITY 6.6   PRACTICAL

Spend some time in front of a mirror and see if you can demonstrate to yourself these feelings with your facial expressions.

As this activity is based on your own observations, there is no outline answer at the end of the chapter.

---

2 Listening attentively

This means actively attending to what is being said and how it is being said. It is listening without making judgements or letting your own perceptions act as a barrier to what is being said by the other person. It requires giving signals that you are actively listening by using appropriate prompts, such as 'mmm', 'I see', 'how interesting' or 'OK', and non-verbal prompts, such as nodding and smiling, and also giving feedback to show that you understand what is being said or conveyed. Active listening enables trusting relationships, rapport, mutual interest and understanding.

ACTIVITY 6.7   PRACTICAL

Arrange two chairs back to back. Have a friend sit on one chair and yourself on the other. Have the friend tell you about a journey they have just taken. Let them speak for a couple of minutes. Do not interrupt your friend or ask any questions. When they have stopped, recount to them what they told you. Then place the chairs facing each other. Sit opposite your friend and ask them to tell you about their day at work for two minutes. Again, do not interrupt or ask questions. When they have finished, relate back to them what they have recounted to you.

Compare the two experiences from two points:

- How did it feel to listen and not speak?
- Did you remember more from the first or the second task about the events?

As this activity is based on your own observations, there is no outline answer at the end of the chapter.

---

3 Interpreting accurately

To begin interpreting information that has been verbalised begins, not by leaping in to form an opinion on what has been said, but with assessing the extent of the other person's level of understanding. It also requires collecting any cues from non-verbal information and assessing the extent of this influence on what has been said. To make this estimation, you will use as your baseline your own experience or level of knowledge and expertise about the situation or condition. It is then possible to make a judgement or evaluation on the accuracy of this understanding, which can then be utilised, for example, to help a patient gain further understanding of health advice on weight management or to improve accuracy of a procedure in the case of a fellow student. Therefore, interpreting means gathering information before you form an explanation of a situation or events with the intention of improving understanding.

Interpreting messages is also a form of translating and you may be called upon to translate from one language to another, such as from bioscientific terms used in medicine into everyday language, to enable understanding or meaningful comprehension. It could also involve taking a complex idea and transforming it into a simpler and more understandable idea that is related to the real-world situation of the patient or setting.

4 Giving clear instructions

This is a skill that requires practice and is harder than it seems. One way to become accomplished is to talk through what you are doing as you are carrying out an activity, and (this is most important) say why you are doing what you are doing.

ACTIVITY 6.8   PRACTICAL

Write down all the steps it takes to make a cup of tea. Then add a reason for each step. Compare the number of steps you take with a friend. Are they the same? Was it easy to give a reason for something you do almost automatically? Most people have their own idiosyncratic way of undertaking a procedure, so that your way of doing something, no matter how simple, is likely to be different from another's. Bear this in mind when you want a person to follow your instructions. Give explanations so that they understand why, in this situation, they are expected to do the activity differently, or find out how they would carry out the procedure and say why it needs to be different, or use their methods if appropriate.

As this activity depends on your own observations, there is no outline answer at the end of the chapter.

Always begin with the simplest explanation and work towards the more complex. This is invaluable when you are carrying out procedures with patients whom you require to participate, but who may be anxious. In these situations gradual exposure to information is needed so that their anxiety is not further increased by unnecessary information and the information should be paced according to their information needs. However, when teaching a skill to colleagues, a different tack is needed whereby all the information will need to be transmitted; yet this can also be in a graded and staged approach to facilitate assimilation and retention of information.

5 Behaving in a professional manner

Nurses have a legal and moral duty to maintain their competency and to work within the scope of their practice. There is an expectation that you will act in a professional manner, and establish realistic boundaries related to time, purpose of the interaction and level of involvement with patients and those in your care. These principles can also relate to interactions with fellow students and colleagues. Intrinsic to these principles are notions of respect for basic human dignity, cultural openness, sensitivity to individuals' circumstances, an understanding of the impact of ill health or disability and adherence to standards of care. Conveying these attributes to your audience and to patients is an important part of demonstrating your professional awareness and competence. A further consideration is the use of research evidence to improve nursing practice, which can be integrated into your educator role through, for example, patient information on health-promoting activities and into informational presentations for colleagues.

6 Communicating information clearly

The first step to clear information is to know your audience and what they will accept as a preferred means for messages to be communicated. Questions to consider are: which language is being used – jargon or lay terms, what dialect (nurses need to switch from one form of language to another in relation to dialect or generation), whether humour is acceptable, whether the messages should be personalised, whether learning styles are an important factor to consider, and whether a different style is required for children, adults with learning difficulties or aggressive patients (covered more specifically elsewhere in this book). When all these factors are considered the appropriate message medium can be selected to transmit the information.

The next step is to decide if the message is task- or relationship-oriented. An example is the instructions given by flight attendants before take-off. If humour is injected to gain your attention, are you annoyed, as you believe it trivialises the information, or does it make you sit up and listen? The task is the information about safety procedures, whereas the relational aspect is the inclusion of personalised remarks that could either reduce tension or create tension. You will have to decide which approach to use by knowing your audience. There will be times when the task is the most important aspect of the communication, perhaps in emergency situations, and there will be other occasions when the relational and more emotional aspects will be paramount. It has to be noted that patient satisfaction with healthcare is most often rated more highly when nurses recognise a person's fears and worries. This can be transmitted succinctly with a few words. Similarly, if students feel their personal needs are recognised, they will respond to information receptively. However, if the patient or colleague is sending out signals that they only want to know the task-related information, then this what is needed.

7 Establishing credibility

As a student, you may believe that you have little credibility as an educator, yet credibility can also equal believability, which is the ability to inspire belief or trust. You may wish to consider how you could demonstrate these characteristics to others in a manner that may not rest solely on your nursing knowledge, but more on the type of person you are or are becoming. In the early stages of your course, you may feel unable to take on the responsibility of teaching others. However, as you progress through the programme, even moving from one year to the next, you will be in a position to help more junior students with advice and information. Credibility is also about your acceptability among your colleagues, and demonstrating that you can be reliable or helpful can generate acceptability. The perception that a person is competent, knowledgeable and skilled enhances credibility. Demonstrating these characteristics in areas where you have proven your ability, such as through examinations or presentations to your colleagues, is particularly effective in strengthening interpersonal relationships.

Student as lifelong learner

The NMC *Standards of Proficiency* (2004a) stress that nurses should commit themselves to lifelong learning, safely and effectively extend the scope of their professional practice and think in a future-directed and nursing branch-related way. However, the idea was first articulated by Basil Yeaxlee and Eduard Lindeman in the

1900s, when education was proposed as a continuing aspect of everyday life. The notion of learning through life is therefore not new and a peep into the Greek philosopher Plato's (428–348 BC) work *Republic* would show the thinking that we do not stop learning in childhood. Initially, lifelong learning was seen as adult learning and was deemed to be for learning's sake and therefore non-vocational. It was seen to build upon existing formal education, to extend beyond formal education providers to groups, such as religious or union groups and societies, and upon a belief that individuals will see the value of education and will therefore become self-directed learners.

A gradual shift has taken place for lifelong education to be reconceptualised as lifelong learning. The world we inhabit has seen economic, social and cultural change, where many live in a 'knowledge' or 'informational' society, which has strong individualised tendencies requiring continual striving to keep up with technologic and societal developments. The result is that adults now take part in many non-formal learning activities, such as short courses, study tours, fitness centres, sports clubs, heritage centres, self-help therapies, consulting management gurus, electronic networks and self-instructional videos.

Career Framework

In 2001, the Department of Health announced proposals for a five-year action plan to encourage lifelong learning opportunities for all levels of staff in the NHS (DH, 2001). The plan was intended to reinforce the importance of learning and personal development for all staff to be linked to patient care and service improvement. This was a clear indicator that staff in the NHS need to continue to develop their knowledge and skills in order to remain current over their lifetime in the organisation, but also to provide a progressive and explicit staged approach to career opportunity and development. This was further explored by the Skills for Health Department, which produced a Career Framework in 2006 (**www.skillsforhealth.org.uk/page/ career-framework**).

The framework has nine levels, each relating to a higher level of seniority and level of skill acquisition. The aim is to provide a guide for NHS and partner organisations on the implementation of a flexible career and skills escalation, thus enabling an individual member of staff to progress in a direction that meets workforce, service and individual needs.

Level 9

More Senior Staff
Staff with the ultimate responsibility for clinical caseload decision making and full on-call accountability.

Level 8

Consultant Practitioners
Staff working at a very high level of clinical expertise and/or having responsibility for planning of services.

Level 7

Advanced Practitioners
Experienced clinical professionals who have developed their skills and theoretical knowledge to a very high standard. They are empowered to make high-level clinical decisions and will often have their own caseload. Non-clinical staff at Level 7 will typically be managing a number of service areas.

Level 6

Senior Practitioners/Specialist Practitioners
Staff who would have a higher degree of autonomy and responsibility than 'Practitioner' in the clinical environment, or who would be managing one or more service areas in the non-clinical environment.

Level 5

Practitioners
Most frequently registered practitioners in their first and second post-registration/professional qualification jobs.

Level 4

Assistant Practitioners/Associate Practitioners
Probably studying for foundation degree, BTEC higher or HND. Some of their remit will involve them in delivering protocol-based clinical care that had previously been in the remit of registered professionals, under the direction and supervision of a state registered practitioner.

Level 3

Senior Healthcare Assistants/Technicians
Have a higher level of responsibility than support workers, probably studying for, or have attained, NVQ level 3, or Assessment of Prior Experiential Learning (APEL).

Level 2

Support Workers
Frequently with the job title of 'Healthcare Assistant' or 'Healthcare Technician'; probably studying for or have attained NVQ level 2.

Level 1

Initial Entry Level Jobs
Such as 'Domestics' or 'Cadets', requiring very little formal education or previous knowledge, skills or experience in delivering, or supporting the delivery of, healthcare.

Importance of skills

The increasing importance of skills in the UK population is seen as a major challenge when set against world economic forecasts for global economies. The emphasis on skills remains key to government objectives, with the findings of the Leitch review of skills being produced by the Treasury in 2007 (**www.hm-treasury.gov.uk/ independent_reviews/leitch_review/review_leitch_index.cfm**). The aim is for the UK to become a world leader in skills to enable the country to compete with the rest of the world. This may seem a lofty ambition, and far removed from your studies as a student nurse. Yet, the implications for you and your future working life are that you will need to be aware of the demographic changes that are impacting qualified practitioners in the health field as well as people in all walks of life.

The UK has a relatively strong economy with, currently, high employment rates. However, we are not in a position to be complacent, as the demand for high-level skills is going to increase as global competition for resources also increases. Our population continues to age, and there are rapid changes in technological developments. We are relying more and more on innovation to drive our economic growth. The ability to do this relies on a nation's skills and knowledge. Currently, our nation's skills are not world class. National productivity trails many of our main international comparators. The UK has high levels of child poverty, poor employment rates for the disadvantaged, regional differences and high income inequality. It is perceived that improving skills levels can reverse these trends.

We do have an excellent HE system, where more people than ever before are studying and where there are good initiatives in vocational training. However, in 2007 more than one third of all adults did not hold a basic school-leaving qualification, almost one half of adults had difficulty with numbers and one seventh were functionally illiterate. The Leitch review recommended a radical change across the skills spectrum and proposed three levels of skills – basic, intermediate and advanced – which will be initiated with the new proposal for skills to be assessed at the age of 14 in schools with the introduction a new diploma qualification.

Your future career path will be guided by many factors, ranging from your personal circumstances to your career goals and aspirations. The Skills for Health Career Framework (see pages 119–20) will provide an outline for you to gauge what further education and learning you will need. Following successful completion of your course, you will enter the framework at level 5. Specialist practitioners are well established in many fields, such as renal nursing and diabetes, and have gained recognition in the Career Framework at level 6. The role of advanced practitioner is not yet fully embedded in nursing practice or recognised within a regulatory framework, but there are many examples of advanced practitioner roles developing in all fields of nursing practice, particularly in primary care, and recognition is given at level 7 to these practitioners. Consultant nurse practitioners at level 8 are fewer in number, but have been established in fields such as intensive care and mental health.

Even if you decide to stay and are comfortable at level 5, there is every likelihood that, due to changes in technology and the moving frontiers of knowledge, you will be required to learn new skills and acquire new knowledge. Indeed, to remain a registered practitioner you will be required meet the NMC standards for continuing registration by completing 35 hours or five days of learning in the previous three years and 450 hours of practice in each area of registration. Lifelong learning will be integral to your continuing professional knowledge and competence. You may also wish to continue to learn and develop areas of knowledge that give you additional interest and pleasure in life. Alongside this will be your continuing development of CIPS at each stage of your professional life.

CHAPTER SUMMARY

In this chapter, we have looked at three stages of learning opportunity for students. Rather than concentrate on the classical approach to study skills, which can be found in excellent resources such as Maslin-Prothero and Taylor (2005) and Taylor (2003), we have taken a path that discusses how students can integrate theory with practice. There is no doubt that learning for reality should be the goal for nursing students as they combine theory with practice. In this chapter, we have suggested that this can be achieved by experiential learning and have provided a model to develop this skill. To enable a clearer understanding of what is expected in academic studies, we have examined academic frameworks and considered how practice can be aligned by utilising the SEEC descriptors. The relevance of reflective learning was established, although there remain concerns that learning styles are an important consideration if reflection is to be effective. Guidance on how to achieve a skilled performance has been provided for skills development. The role of a student as educator was explored, and guidance has been given for achieving effective communication in healthcare settings. Finally, the relevance of lifelong learning, both personal and professional, has been examined and we have given brief consideration to future career possibilities following completion of the course.

Activities: brief outline answers

As the results of all the activities in this chapter are based on your own observations and decision-making abilities, there are no outline answers for this chapter.

KNOWLEDGE REVIEW

Having completed the chapter, how would you now rate your knowledge of the following topics?

	Good	Adequate	Poor
1. Integration of theory and practice.			
2. Reflective writing.			
3. Health communication skills.			
4. Lifelong learning.			

Where you're not confident in your knowledge of a topic, what will you do next?

Further reading

Arnold, E. and Boggs, KU (2004) *Interpersonal Relationships: Professional communication skills for nurses*. London: Elsevier.

Maslin-Prothero, S (ed.) (2005) *Bailliere's Study Skills for Nurses and Midwives*. Oxford: Bailliere Tindall.

Quinn, F and Hughes, S (2007) *Quinn's Principles and Practice of Nurse Education*. Oxford: Nelson Thornes.

Rolfe, G, Freshwater, D and Jasper, M. (2001) *Critical Reflection for Nursing and the Helping Professions: A user's guide*. Basingstoke: Palgrave.

Taylor, J (2003) *Foundations in Nursing and Health Care: Study skills in health care*. Cheltenham: Nelson Thornes.

Useful websites

www.businessballs.com/kolblearningstyles.htm This site has details on Kolb's learning styles inventory, and a brief comparison with Honey and Mumford's variation on the theory.

www.campaign-for-learning.org.uk/cfl/yourlearning/whatlearner.asp This has details on Honey and Mumford's learning styles inventory; it provides an outline of the four styles and suggestions for your preferred learning methods.

www.qaa.ac.uk/academicinfrastructure/default.asp This site has details of the academic qualifications framework.

www.qaa.ac.uk/students/guides/UnderstandQuals.asp The Understanding Qualifications website has the frameworks for HE qualifications.

www.skillsforhealth.org.uk This is the Skills for Health Department, which produced a Career Framework.

7. The environmental context

CHAPTER AIMS

After reading this chapter, you will be able to:

- understand how different care settings might undermine the practice of safe and effective communication and interpersonal skills (CIPS);

- describe the importance of physical and social environmental factors on the practice of good communication in healthcare and be able to identify examples of each, in relation to communication within groups or families and between younger and older people;

- understand what is meant by the terms 'prejudice' and 'schema development' and their relation to language use in nursing;

- appreciate the demands on CIPS in British nursing placed by the nature of multiculturalism;

- identify the ways in which institutional racism impact on communication and interpersonal exchanges in British nursing practice and the ways in which healthcare organisations defend themselves from accepting that they may be institutionally racist;

- know what is meant by 'cultural competence', 'cultural awareness' and 'transcultural nursing care';

- describe the meaning of the 'fallacy of individualism' as it pertains to CIPS practice in British nursing care.

Introduction

The environmental context of communication and interpersonal skills (CIPS) for nurses includes multidisciplinary team practice and interprofessional working, across different care settings, within a safe environment. The *Concise Oxford Dictionary of Current English* (Thompson, 1995) defines 'safety' in two ways, one positive and one negative: first, as *free of danger or injury; affording security* and being *free of harm*; second, in terms of being cautious, unenterprising and consistently moderate.

The first way of defining safety seems both helpful and non-contentious. The second, however, might speak to the use of 'safety in practice' in anti-therapeutic, risk-averse ways, which can undermine the deployment of good CIPS (see the section below entitled 'A specific environmental example: endless rows of chairs' in illustration of this point). Clearly, different care settings will either promote or undermine the concept of 'safe environments'.

With the above in mind, this chapter will begin by introducing you to a discussion on the importance of CIPS within multidisciplinary team practice and interprofessional working, across different care settings, within a safe environment. A specific case study will be presented of sexual abuse within a care home. This case study is intended to help you recognise the relationship between a lack of safety and a breakdown in communication within a specific care environment.

The discussion will then turn to the ways in which physical and social environmental factors are key to shaping communication, and this will be illustrated with the ways in which the physical environment of nursing care can undermine the possibilities for good communication. With regard to the social environment, communication within groups and families, and between young and older people, will be discussed and illustrated with appropriate examples.

Next, we will help you explore the interrelated concepts of prejudice and schema development. These concepts (introduced in Chapter 3) have emerged from developmental psychology and, together with the role of language use, are extremely important in understanding how CIPS can break down in specific healthcare environmental contexts.

The next topic to be discussed will be that of how shifting friendship, family and cultural networks impact on communication and interpersonal behaviour and skill development. The demands on CIPS arising from British multicultural society will then be contrasted with institutional racism, and its impact on communication, in healthcare environments. To combat such racism, the important skill of 'cultural competence' and its relationship to **transcultural** healthcare will be discussed.

The chapter will end with a critique of the tendency emerging from humanistic psychology to view CIPS as solely located within the individual. In the light of the preceding argument, this 'fallacy of **individualism**' will be seen to both be naive and convey an overly optimistic picture of human interaction.

Multidisciplinary team practice and interprofessional working

The demands of two or more professional groups communicating effectively within the same team are considerable. When environmental factors are added to the melting pot, the recipe for danger can increase in an alarming way. The following case study demonstrates a specific example of a phenomenon prevalent in recent years, and makes for disturbing reading.

CASE STUDY

Sexual abuse of the elderly in relation to communication

On 25 February 2001, *The Guardian* newspaper reported an example of the sexual abuse of an elderly woman in a nursing home. In 1991, she suddenly stopped taking her medication. At that time, her family made the assumption that this behaviour was related to an inevitable progression of her slide towards Alzheimer's that had begun some years earlier. However, soon afterwards, she exhibited terror each time her formerly beloved son-in-law entered her room at her nursing home. Again, her family made sense of this in terms of her illness progressing very quickly.

It was only when the owner of the nursing home was arrested for sexual attacks on the elderly women in his care that the family began to piece together a number of strange incidents that had escaped their notice at the time. At that point the old lady had since died. Her daughter was of the opinion that her mother wasn't listed as a victim in the court case because the authorities didn't seem to want to go into it. She further asserted that none of the children whose mothers were abused in the home knew what was going on.

The owner of the nursing home – a man in his mid-sixties – was sentenced to four years in jail. That was in 1997. But the probability is that the sexual abuse of old people by care workers is still going on today and could be as common as that suffered by children in the days before the paedophile problem was recognised.

Some years later, the Director of the website and helpline, Action on Elder Abuse (www.elderabuse.org.uk), expressed the view that sexual abuse of elderly people in care and nursing homes was extremely prevalent. She stated that the helpline received lots of calls from frantic families and care home staff concerning extreme sexual abuse in these homes, and was of the opinion that the number of calls grossly under-represented the true level of abuse taking place. She gave the view that someone suffering from mental and physical frailty was the perfect victim for such abuse, given that they can't defend themselves or get away from the environment they find themselves in.

She added that, in her view, such abuse was more about power than sex, and that there were even pages on paedophile websites encouraging men finding it hard to access children to gain employment at care homes.

Catalogue of assault

According to the Action on Elder Abuse handbook, there are five main types of abuse in care homes.

- **Physical** – includes hitting and restraining, or giving too much, or the wrong, medication.
- **Psychological** – shouting, swearing, frightening or humiliating a person.
- **Financial** – illegal or unauthorised use of a person's property, money, pension book or other valuables.
- **Sexual** – forcing a person to take part in any sexual activity without his or her consent.
- **Neglect** – where a person is deprived of food, heat, clothing, comfort or essential medication.

The environmental impact on communication

The importance of environmental factors in skilled interpersonal communication was argued in Chapter 3 (Hargie and Dickson, 2004). To recapitulate, Hargie and Dickson argued the crucial relevance of the 'person-situation' context for making sense of interpersonal communication. Hendricks and Hendricks (1986) supported this standpoint from the perspective of social-environmental theory, which emphasises the environment as a very important factor in shaping communication. With regard to the elderly, for example, the residential healthcare environment produces both opportunities and constraints between staff and patients/clients, generally and specifically, around communication. As can be seen from the above worst-case scenario of sexual abuse, communication between staff and patients, and between patients and their relatives, can be seriously compromised under conditions of extreme exploitation of patients.

The physical environment

The 'environment' in this theory is defined as both physical and social. At a physical environmental level, the layout and shape of the building can both provide opportunity for, and constrain, good interpersonal communication. In illustration of this, Nussbaum et al. argue that:

> the architectural design of a nursing home can 'control' the interaction within the building. If the nursing home is designed with a central nursing station and has residential wings extending from the center, it is very unlikely that individuals who are placed in separate wings will enter into a relationship. Proximity is a primary factor for selecting an individual for interaction, and the architecture often dictates who will be close both physically and relationally.

(2000, p14)

environment that enable good communication between healthcare workers and patients/clients. In the other, list the aspects that inhibit or undermine the possibility of such good communication.

As this activity is based on your own observations, there is no outline answer at the end of the chapter.

A specific environmental example: endless rows of chairs

The second author spent some time in the early 1980s as a charge nurse in an acute unit for mentally ill older people. Throughout his nurse training, he had noticed the tendency of chairs on ward dayrooms, especially on wards for older people, to be in a row against the dayroom walls. In his view, also expressed by many other nurse writers and practitioners at the time, this reinforced isolation and prevented communication among patients/clients.

ACTIVITY 7.3   PRACTICAL

With your student colleagues, try sitting in a row of chairs as described above. Note how this affects communication between you all and list these after a group discussion of the experience.

As this activity is based on your own observations, there is no outline answer at the end of the chapter.

In the second author's first few days in charge of the acute unit, he imagined he had the power to make environmental changes to improve communication by changing the position of the chairs in the dayroom to allow for, rather than inhibit, communication among the patients. The chairs were arranged in small circles of four and the intention was to keep them this way and observe for any increase in communication between the patients. When he next came back on shift he noticed, to his dismay and irritation, that the chairs had been moved back to their original position in rows against each wall. Once again, he had them moved back into small circles of four, but each time he went off duty they were moved back against the wall.

This rearrangement of the chairs went on for several days until he found out that the ward cleaners, with the blessing of their managers, had been moving them back to their original positions to ease their cleaning duties. He found his own, nursing, management unsupportive of his idea of moving chairs to improve communication on 'health and safety' grounds ('the patients might trip over the chairs'). This example of a failed experiment aimed to improve communication between patients clearly illustrates the double-sided nature of safety mentioned in the introduction to this chapter. Questions arise as to who wins and who loses in this picture of chairs placed in rows in the interest of 'safety'.

The social environment

Communication within groups and families will vary in style, content and function. Researchers working in the related areas of social identity theory (SIT) and self-categorisation theory (SCT) argue that group norms influence behaviour when the social identities with which they are associated are meaningful to the individuals in the group (Augoustinos et al., 2006). Put more simply, people in different social groups or families will experience social identities that 'work' precisely because other members in their particular group or family experience themselves as having similar or complementary social identities.

Social identities will correspond to specific sets of attitudes, behaviour and communication styles, and to **culture** and **ethnicity** (to be discussed in Chapter 8). Possible implications emerging from this knowledge base include the difficulties individuals may have in communicating if they are removed from their usual social context. Their ability to adapt to their new circumstances is likely to depend on the flexibility of their personal schemas (see Chapter 3) and their mastery of the language used in the new social environment they find themselves in (see discussion on both of these topics below); their age; their perception of how safe they feel; and perhaps numerous other factors.

ACTIVITY 7.4   REFLECTIVE

In a group, discuss times when you felt uncomfortable in strange environments (for example if you were admitted to hospital as a young child). What things helped and what things made you feel worse? Can you relate either the things that helped or made you feel worse to specific aspects of interpersonal contact and communication?

As this activity is based on your own reflection, there is no outline answer at the end of the chapter.

Communication between young and older persons

Given the findings of SIT and SCT, interpersonal communication within the social environment will be influenced by differences between what is taken for granted in nursing and client cultures with regard to speech. This will, in turn, be affected by generational and ethnic differences both within and between these groups.

Some key issues of interpersonal communication between nurses and patients/clients from different ethnic groups will be discussed later in this chapter. For the moment, consider the ways in which differences in speech and language, and overall communication, between, for example, young and older people can often be marked. Younger nurses may take for granted the way that they speak, and dress, as right and proper, without considering the offence they may cause directly or indirectly to their patients/clients. Consider a contemporary case study about nursery staff deriving from Matt Lucas's character 'Vicky Pollard' in *Little Britain*.

CASE STUDY

Nurses as 'Vicky Pollards'

In the *Daily Mail*, on 16 December 2007, the Chair of the Professional Association of Teachers described the dangers of illiterate nursery staff who discuss their social lives in front of toddlers and who adopt inappropriate communication and dress styles. She said that too many students starting childcare training courses write using only the shorthand language of text messages. She also argued that growing numbers of young staff in nurseries dress inappropriately, with long nails and 'chunky' shoes, and inappropriately discussed their nights out drinking in front of children.

This teaching expert had nearly 30 years' experience of working in education, including inspecting playgroups and nurseries. She argued that those training to be nursery workers are acting as role models for children and are in danger of creating a generation of 'Vicky Pollards'.

ACTIVITY 7.5   **REFLECTIVE**

In small groups, discuss the implications of the above press report for nurses in relation to particular patient/client groups, for example the elderly, children's nursing, or nurses visiting families.

As this activity is based on your own reflection and discussions, there is no outline answer at the end of the chapter.

'Baby talk' and caring for the elderly

How representative Vicky Pollard is of the younger generation of nurses is an interesting question. However, the case study above demonstrates the importance of the social environmental communication context for nursing practice and how easily this can be ethically and professionally violated because of the unquestioned dress and behaviour code of some employees. Another stark example of nurses not paying sufficient attention to the person-situation context is in the use of what has been described as 'baby talk'.

Ryan and Hamilton (1994) studied nurse–patient interactions with elderly nursing home residents. Some nurses demonstrate a lack of respect in their use of baby talk, and related voice tone and parental style. Nurses and volunteers using baby talk were rated less respectful and competent than their peers and elderly recipients of such baby talk were, clearly understandably, less satisfied with the interaction.

The use of baby talk and 'Vicky Pollard' behaviour raises interesting questions about how many healthcare workers, including nurses, take for granted the assumptions they have about themselves, and the world and others within it. These questions alert us to the need to be mindful of how such assumptions develop.

Prejudice and schema development

None of us is born with psychological maps or templates for understanding the world, other people or ourselves. These develop over time, mostly in childhood, as a result of our interactions in the world with significant others, particularly our parent or parents. Described as *schemas*, or *core beliefs* (Grant et al., 2004), these are necessary to equip us to make sense of ourselves in interaction with others and in changing life circumstances and situations.

Those of us fortunate enough to have good enough parenting will develop schemas (see Chapter 3), which enable us to get by reasonably successfully in the world, and with other people and ourselves. However, equally, because of abusive early life experiences, many of us will grow up with a core sense of ourselves as 'worthless', 'bad', 'useless' or something equally self-denigrating.

VIEWING SCHEMAS AS 'SELF-PREJUDICE'

In her ground-breaking work on helping the kind of people described immediately above, Padesky (1991) explains how she helps clients begin to consider how their deeply held negative schemas are a form of 'self-prejudice'. She does this by asking clients to bring to mind someone in their life who is deeply prejudiced. This prejudice may, for example, be directed towards certain groups of people because of their religious or sexual orientation. She then engages in a dialogue with them to help them review the ways in which such prejudices may be maintained through forms of selective information processing. This can include attending to information that confirms the 'truth' of the prejudice, while ignoring or discounting evidence that challenges it. Clients are then invited to consider the similarities between their own deeply held negative schemas and the prejudices and prejudiced people they have been discussing.

ACTIVITY 7.6   PRACTICAL

Log on to **www.padesky.com**. From there, follow the links to 'Clinical Corner' and left click on 'Publications'. In this page you will find Padesky's article 'Schema as prejudice'. Read this article and discuss it in small groups in your class. Consider possible implications for interpersonal communication in your work as a nurse.

As this activity is based on your own reflection and discussions, there is no outline answer at the end of the chapter.

A strikingly ironic feature of deeply held prejudices, whether – in Padesky's terms – they are prejudices held against oneself or directed towards societal groups, is that they are often not experienced by the people who hold them as prejudices at all! Instead, they are considered to be right and proper, and common sense – a reflection of the world as it is, rather than a distortion of reality or a bigoted point of view. In order for someone to begin to rid themselves of their prejudice/s, they would have to begin to question them and see them as contingent (dependent on events and circumstances in their upbringing) rather than absolutely true.

It may be helpful at this stage to consider the extent to which we all hold beliefs and assumptions about our life-worlds that remain taken for granted as 'just so' rather than potentially or actually problematic.

NURSING AND DOMINANT CULTURAL BELIEFS

It has been suggested that a majority of nursing is delivered from the value position of [nurses], which may be based on their dominant cultural beliefs (Parfitt, 1998). Ironically, the vast majority of indigenous healthcare workers have rarely, if ever, previously given consideration as to what their values and cultural beliefs are. Or how their values, beliefs and cultural traditions are acquired. Yet most assume, with equal measures of ignorance and arrogance, that their 'British' culture is the right way and that it is naturally superior to all other 'uncivilised or unsophisticated' cultures. Regrettably, those who possess that chauvinistic attitude will come into conflict with patients/clients who are not Anglicized or 'British'. That negative tension or cultural conflict, if not rapidly dispelled, will ultimately undermine the therapeutic relationship between patient and [nurse]; and therefore the quality of care will be compromised.

(Narayanasamy and White, 2005, p104)

Padesky, and other cognitive psychotherapy writers (Grant et al., 2004, 2008; Hayes and Smith, 2005) argue that prejudices and other forms of deeply held belief are maintained through engaging in speech and language, and related behaviour, which give form and substance to the prejudice. In this regard, there are two interesting views of the world that may be useful to contemplate: in the first, the world is more or less separate from the language we use to describe it; in the second, the world is constituted or given shape, substance and reality by language.

THEORY SUMMARY

The Sapir–Whorf hypothesis

That language defines the way a person behaves and thinks was argued by Edward Sapir (1983) and his student and colleague Benjamin Whorf (1956). Both believed that language and the thoughts that we have are somehow interwoven, and that all people are equally affected by the confines of their language. In short, they argued that all people are in a sense mental prisoners, unable to think freely because of the restrictions of their vocabularies.

An example of this idea is apparent in George Orwell's famous book *1984*, in which he discusses the use of a language he calls 'newspeak', which was developed to change the way people thought about the government. The new vocabulary they were given was created to control their minds. Since they could not think of things not included in the vocabulary, they were, by default, zombies, imprisoned by the trance of their language. Sapir and Whorf coined the term 'linguistic determinism' to capture the notion of ideas and creativity as the prisoners of vocabulary. If people indeed cannot think outside the confines of their language, the result of this process is many different world-views by speakers of different languages.

According to Sapir and Whorf, an idea complementary to linguistic determinism is 'linguistic relativity', which states that the differences in language reflect the different views of people from different cultures.

It follows from the above that, if the world-view and behaviour of people are affected so severely by the structure of their language, and languages have different structures, then is cross-cultural communication and understanding a realistic possibility in the modern world? The Sapir–Whorf hypothesis would have us believe that such barrier-free communication is almost impossible. There is no question that the vocabulary of a specific language mirrors whatever the non-verbal culture emphasises. For example, aspects of the society that are not associated directly with language seem to have a direct impact on the formation of language. A society where horses are revered will have many words for horses and horse-related things – not because horses talk, but because people talk about their horses. Important parts of a society are certainly highlighted in the vocabulary of a language. For example, the Eskimos may have many words for snow, the Americans for cars and the Norwegians for fish. But this does not necessarily mean that other cultures are incapable of perceiving the items that are described with such specific vocabulary elsewhere.

In criticism of the Sapir–Whorf hypothesis, if the English language was somehow keeping us from freedom of thought, we would all be trapped in the same cognitive path if we were English speakers. However, even among siblings, the understanding of certain words and what they mean varies. This is due to different environmental factors, personal interests, friends and teachers, and perhaps an age difference. Two people who live in the same house, with the same genetic make-up and speaking the same language should have the same cognitive processes if we were prisoners of our language. We are obviously not. However, awareness of, and discussion around, the Sapir–Whorf hypothesis are important parts of globalisation, communication and cultural education in the world today.

If the Sapir–Whorf hypothesis is accepted to a greater or lesser extent, the degree to which we are all more or less 'trapped within' language in making sense of, and constructing, our worlds has fairly clear implications for nursing people from different cultures. For example, something that one cultural group takes for granted, in relation to healthcare and communication, may be alien and experienced as deeply strange by another group. This is made all the more complex by the fact that, within one culture, there may be many, shifting and evolving, subcultures. Wikipedia defines a 'subculture' as *a group of people with a set of behaviors and beliefs that could be distinct or hidden, and which differentiate them from the larger culture to which they belong*.

Shifting friendship, family and cultural networks

In was argued above (Augoustinos et al., 2006), on the basis of SIT and SCT, that social identity is experienced in relation to the primary reference group that a person belongs to, be it family and/or friends or colleagues. Within the space of a lifetime, an individual is likely to shift primary reference groups several, perhaps many, times and develop identities and related values and communication styles different from, and possibly in opposition to, their families and original reference groups.

Such shifts may be radical in form. For example, the 1960s saw the emergence of 'Flower Power' and Psychedelia. Ten years later, the Punk movement emerged, partly in reaction against the music, style, attitudes and forms of communication associated with Psychedelia. Both Psychedelia and the Punk movement could be described as subcultures. Subcultures exist in opposition, or run counter, to the dominant culture within which they are embedded. Thus, according to Wikipedia, they effectively exist to disrupt the dominant culture, as a '**counterculture**'.

Within Britain, in addition to sub- and countercultures, shifting populations with their different health needs – for example, refugees – are currently moving within and between changing social contexts such as family structures and friendship networks. In regard to ethnic differences alone, this gives rise to a rich and complex multicultural picture, which has clear implications for the need for skilled interpersonal communication, and related awareness, among nurses.

Institutional racism

Insensitive behaviour to people from different ethnic groups, whether it results from deeply held prejudices, ignorance or simply thoughtlessness, can often produce an organisational picture of institutional racism.

CASE STUDY

The Macpherson Report (1999) suggested that most of Britain's public institutions displayed institutional racism, defined as:

> *The collective failure of an organisation to provide an appropriate and professional service to people because of their colour, culture or ethnic origin. It can be seen or detected in processes, attitudes and behaviour which amount to discrimination through unwitting prejudice, ignorance, thoughtlessness and racist stereotyping which disadvantage minority ethnic people.*

(Macpherson, 1999, p10)

CASE STUDY

Google 'Rocky Bennett Inquiry' and read the websites that come up. In October 1998, David 'Rocky' Bennett died as a result of forced restraint by up to five nurses at the Norvic Clinic psychiatric in-patient unit. Preceding this event, he was the victim of sustained institutional racism by both staff and clients alike. Narayanasamy and White (2005) assert the belief that institutional racism pervades healthcare, including nursing. It certainly seems to be the case that Rocky Bennett was the tragic victim of this problem, but how representative of a more general trend is this? One thing's for sure: ask many nurses if it goes on in their workplace and they'll deny it. This kind of response represents a kind of defensive 'NIMBYism' (not in my back yard) that should alert the enquirer to the possible operation of organisational defence mechanisms (Morgan, 1997).

Developing the propositions of psychoanalyst Sigmund Freud, Morgan (1997) argued that organisations, in terms of their collective worker mindset, are just like individuals in using unconscious protective measures to escape blame. Table 7.1 (adapted from Grant et al., 2004) illustrates this argument in relation to institutional racism and related interpersonal communication difficulties.

According to Morgan (1997), organisational defence mechanisms, by definition, occur at an organisationally unconscious level. In relation to this, because healthcare organisations have a tendency to socialise many of their members into a 'silent and tacit' agreement with the organisation's values and 'the way things are done around here', nurses may relatively rapidly forget the idealism they had when training in favour of buying into the kinds or organisational communication styles and difficulties described above.

Table 7.1: Organisational defence mechanisms.

Defence mechanism	Defence mechanism defined	Possible communication difficulties
Repression	Pushing unacceptable ideas and impulses into the unconscious.	The possibility that abuse and communication neglect goes on in our organisation is relegated to the organisational unconscious.
Denial	Refusing to acknowledge a disturbing fact, feeling or memory.	Presenting a public face of transculturalism while maintaining institutionally racist forms of communication and refusing to acknowledge this at an organisational level.
Displacement	Shifting disturbing feelings aroused by one person on to a safer target.	Maintaining that 'it is not our responsibility to display culturally sensitive forms of communication because we have not been trained in it'.
Rationalisation	The creation of elaborate or unconvincing schemes of justification to disguise underlying motives and intentions.	Racism does not go on in our organisation. Difficulties in communication between nurses and ethnic minority patient groups are due to circumstances outside our control, including the failure of those patient groups to adapt sufficiently to take advantage of the care on offer.
Regression	Adopting behavioural patterns found satisfying and effective in childhood in order to reduce the effect of uncomfortable demands.	Sending ethnic clients 'to Coventry', by avoiding them and avoiding talking with them.
Splitting and idealisation	Inappropriately separating different elements of experience, and talking up the good aspects of a situation to avoid facing the bad ones.	We represent a centre of excellence in many aspects of our care and this has been acknowledged by feedback from many patients and articles in the local press.

The fallacy of individualism

A difficult but necessary question to pose is to what extent mainstream approaches to the dissemination of CIPS in nursing are embedded in cultural values. A criticism of the widespread reliance on counselling models of interpersonal communication to inform interpersonal skills books in nursing has already been mentioned in Chapter 3 (Brown et al., 2006). Developing this argument from the position of **ethnocentrism**, it can be argued that Rogerian influences (see pages 47–50) in CIPS in nursing betray the assumption of a taken-for-granted individualism.

From an individualistic position, patients/clients and nurses are assumed to have the innate psychological ability to have the power to find their own solutions to their problems, independent of cultural or organisational constraining factors. This includes being able to speak more effectively and genuinely through communication facilitated by the Rogerian core conditions.

What is ignored in the individualistic stance is the fact that environmental, organisational and cultural factors both shape and limit what can be done and said in any interpersonal exchange among nurses, between nurses and other healthcare workers, and between nurses and patients/clients.

Derived from selective aspects of humanistic psychology generally (Whitton, 2003) and Rogerian counselling more specifically (Rogers, 2002), a simple, naive and overly optimistic picture of human interaction emerges. This is about two or more individuals interacting in a cultural and organisational-environmental vacuum.

The humanistic picture of interaction in Figure 7.1 both contrasts with and masks a more challenging image of the nurse and patient/client interacting within multiple cultural and organisational-environmental contexts, which have the power to shape and limit what can be said and done in the name of 'communication and interpersonal skills in nursing' (see Figure 7.2).

Figure 7.1: Simple picture of interaction.

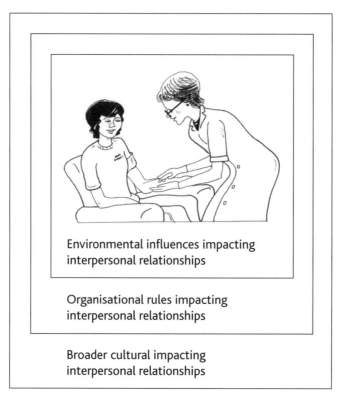

Environmental influences impacting
interpersonal relationships

Organisational rules impacting
interpersonal relationships

Broader cultural impacting
interpersonal relationships

Figure 7.2: Complex picture of interaction.

The individualist/counselling model of skilled communication

There is no such thing as society.

(Margaret Thatcher, 1987)

By placing sole responsibility for good CIPS on nurses, the organisation is let 'off the hook' for the kinds of environmental factors, described above, that work to undermine good communication (Grant, 2002). At a local cultural level, the kinds of unwritten rules, also described above, that result from socialisation into the organisational level, impact communication styles (Morgan, 1997). These rules will affect the quantity and quality of communication between different professional groups and between health workers, including nurses, and patients/clients.

Task, rather than holistic client/patient, workplace cultures will result in 'I–It' rather than 'I–Thou' relationships (see Buber (1958), Chapter 2, pages 34–5). At a broader cultural level, institutional racism and cultural incompetence, and the prejudice that accompanies these problems, are often likely to influence the quality and quantity of nurse–client/patient interpersonal communication, but, unfortunately, remain underacknowledged or denied.

CHAPTER SUMMARY

Different care settings might undermine the practice of safe and effective CIPS. Physical and social environmental factors are very important with regard to the practice of good communication in healthcare, in relation to communication both within groups or families, and between younger and older people. 'Prejudice' and 'schema development', and their relation to language use, are key to understanding examples of poor CIPS in nursing practice. Multiculturalism places demands on CIPS in British nursing, while institutional racism impacts on communication and interpersonal exchanges in British nursing practice. There is a variety of ways in which healthcare organisations defend themselves from accepting that they may be institutionally racist. 'Cultural competence', 'cultural awareness' and 'transcultural nursing care' are crucial skills relating to good communication in British nursing practice. Finally, the 'fallacy of individualism' in CIPS practice in British nursing care masks the important role of environmental, organisational and broader cultural influences impacting such care.

KNOWLEDGE REVIEW

Having completed the chapter, how would you now rate your knowledge of the following topics?

	Good	Adequate	Poor
1. The ways in which different care settings might enhance or undermine good communication among nurses.			
2. How prejudice and schema development influence communication among nurses.			
3. The ways in which transcultural nursing, cultural awareness and competence impact communication skills in nursing.			

Where you're not confident in your knowledge of a topic, what will you do next?

Further reading

Cioffi, J (2006) Culturally diverse patient–nurse interactions on acute care wards. *International Journal of Nursing Practice*, 12(6): 319–25.

Leininger, M (1997) Transcultural nursing research to nursing education and practice: 40 years. *Image Journal of Nursing Scholarship*, 29(4): 341–7.
One hundred culture-specific studies by Leininger.

Nussbaum, JF, Pecchioni, LL, Robinson, JD and Thompson, TL (2000) *Communication and Aging*, 2nd edition. Mahwah, NJ: Lawrence Erlbaum Associates.
As the titles of the above references suggest, you will engage in research on transcultural nursing practices and on communication both between and with elderly clients.

Useful websites

www.elderabuse.org.uk This is a national resource on the issue of abuse of the elderly in care and nursing homes.

www.qmul.ac.uk/news/newsrelease.php?news_id=98 This website discusses research showing institutional racism in the delivery of mental health services to ethnic groups.

8. Population and diversity contexts

CHAPTER AIMS

After reading this chapter, you will be able to:

- understand diversity from different perspectives;
- consider the needs and diversity of populations and individuals within them;
- recognise that care must be respectful and anti-discriminatory;
- understand the need for equity and fairness;
- explore ethical and moral issues in communicating with diverse groups in healthcare settings.

Introduction

Society today is enriched by multicultural, ethnic and social diversity. The focus of this chapter will be on the interpersonal and ethical contexts of nursing people from different backgrounds and cultures. By looking at how populations have evolved in the UK, we will begin by studying the statistical data on **immigration** and **migration** to help understand how diverse ethnic populations in many of our neighbourhoods have developed. We will also explore the motivators behind human migration.

The chapter then divides into two sections, with one focusing on cultures and the next on diversity. Beginning with cultures, we will take into account the range we experience in nursing and the differences that make up a society of diverse groups and identities. Culture is a sociological concept and we will be investigating some of this terrain to gain a deeper understanding of the diversity (the differences between people) and the potential for discrimination. We will concentrate on communicating with cultural diversity by exploring concepts such as cultural preservation, negotiation and repatterning, or restructuring. These are interventions that are geared to changing previously held patterns of behaviour that can have a major detrimental effect on patients' lives and are linked to discriminatory practices.

We explore some of the issues of nursing in a multicultural Britain and the need for cultural awareness and cultural competence, and we compare two theories of transcultural care.

The chapter goes on to examine diversity and socio-economic position, as well as taking time to explore and understand diversity in a society that is made up of different groups to which power, influence and opportunities are not always equally granted. This section briefly discusses race and culture, gender issues, sexual orientation, age and disability.

We will conclude with a section that considers the ethical and moral consequences of communication and personal interactions.

Populations and diversity

From the earliest of times, the islands that make up the United Kingdom (UK) have been settled or invaded by many different peoples: Romans, Saxons, Goths, Vikings and Normans. In more recent times, we have seen, as a result of the two world wars in the last century and the harmonisation policies of the European Union (EU) in this century, people from Europe finding sanctuary, work and education in the UK.

ACTIVITY 8.1   **REFLECTIVE**

Using a range of different sources (e.g. local and national newspapers, magazines, television serials or 'soaps'), make a simple analysis of their portrayal and coverage of peoples of different gender, age, ethnicity and/or religion. Reflect on any differences between local and national media representations. How are messages communicated about culture and diversity in these media? Are there any specific references to culture and diversity and healthcare, and how do they relate to your experiences so far in practice settings?

As this activity is based on your own observations, there is no outline answer at the end of the chapter.

The UK has a history of colonialism – a policy of acquiring land for exploitation and trade that broadened the economic reaches of the UK and set up administration systems in many countries around the globe. This in turn established a network of trade, migration and immigration opportunities that led to the UK recruiting colonial subjects in the Second World War as soldiers; it also recruited men from the Caribbean to work in munitions factories and in Scottish forests. After the war, the UK continued to recruit from the West Indies and Commonwealth countries to meet labour shortages in transport and in the NHS. Links with Africa, Asia and the Far East have also developed immigration routes to the UK and people have settled, bringing with them their cultural practices, traditions, customs, religious beliefs and attitudes, thus providing a rich multicultural tapestry.

ACTIVITY 8.2   **PRACTICAL**

Produce a restaurant menu to reflect the multicultural society of the UK. Remember to consider and include religious and cultural traditions when selecting

---

each dish. How many different dishes did you include? Compare your menu with a fellow student – do you reflect the same cultural differences in your menus? What will you do to find out about the different ethnic groups that make up the diverse population in the UK?

As this activity is based on your own observations, there is no outline answer at the end of the chapter.

Motivation for migrating

Adventurous nomadic groups and individuals, conquering armies and traders of every kind have migrated across the globe for centuries to seek new opportunities, employment and ways of thinking. Consequently, almost all nation states are the product of multiple, overlapping generations of immigrants, not only the UK. It is helpful to understand the motivation behind people's reasons for migrating and these can be classified into different categories.

- Settlers – These are people who intend to live permanently in a new country, mostly in the main countries of settlement such as the United States of America, Canada, Australia and New Zealand. To be a settler you need to qualify in some way and being a skills immigrant, or already having family in the country are usually the main criteria.

- Contract workers – These are admitted to other countries on the understanding that they will stay only a short time. Many are seasonal workers in the agricultural industry. Included in this category are nurses from the Philippines and Eire who are contracted to work in the NHS for short periods. It also includes students attending universities. In nursing, this currently only refers to post-qualifying studies, as the NMC states that only UK citizens can qualify for NMC-regulated pre-registration courses conducted in the UK.

- Professionals – These are people who are employees of transnational companies and who are moved from one country to another. All industrial countries have a system of work permits that regulates the time and scale of residency.

- Undocumented workers – This is a polite term for illegal immigrants. Some have been smuggled into the country and others may have stayed beyond the ends of their work permits.

- Refugees and asylum seekers – A refugee is defined by the United Nations (UN) as someone who has well-founded fear of persecution for reasons of race, religion, nationality, membership of a particular social group or political opinion. During the 1990s, more and more receiving governments started referring to such people as 'asylum seekers' and only termed them 'refugees' when their claims were accepted.

These categories are not exhaustive and do overlap as an Indian medical practitioner working in an NHS hospital may be both a professional and a contract worker.

Data on immigration and migration

You may already be aware that, in England and Wales, a census is undertaken every ten years to survey all people and households in the country. It provides essential information from national to neighbourhood levels for government, business and the community. Data is also collected on immigration and migration and collated by the Office for National Statistics (ONS) (see 'Useful websites' at the end of this chapter). Being informed with accurate data on the reasons why populations migrate and the extent of migration into the UK can not only help nurses understand the reason why people move from one country to another, but also reduce the myths and prejudices that sometimes lie behind beliefs held about immigrants and asylum seekers.

For example, the latest census estimates show that, in the year to mid-2005, a total of 368,000 visits of between one and 12 months were made by overseas residents to England and Wales for work or study purposes: 175,000 for work and 193,000 for study.

The most common non-British country of citizenship for migrants entering the UK in 2005/6 was Poland, whereas, in recent years, India has been the most common. The census shows that Poland and India between them accounted for 24 per cent of non-British migrants entering the UK. Over the same time, Poland became the tenth most common country of citizenship for migrants leaving the UK, indicating a great deal of movement in this group. In 2005/6, British citizens were the largest group of migrants (15 per cent) to arrive in the UK and accounted for more than half of those persons leaving, indicating movement of citizens from the Commonwealth and previous British Protectorates.

Australia was the most popular country of next residence for emigrants and the majority (72 per cent) of emigrants intended to leave the UK for more than four years. In 2006, just 6 per cent of people leaving the UK were of retirement age, whereas only 1 per cent of people entering the UK were in this age group. This indicates a larger exodus of retirees than entrants; however, a larger proportion of emigrants were of working age, indicating a potential loss of skills for the UK.

Home Office releases for 2007/8 show that there were 24,345 applications for asylum, excluding dependants, which was a 7 per cent decrease from 2006/7. This is the second lowest figure for a financial year since 1993/4, following the lowest year in 2006/7. The number of applications for asylum was 16 per cent higher in 2008 than in 2007.

ACTIVITY 8.3   PRACTICAL

You might want to explore the data for yourself and the web addresses can be found at the end of this chapter. If you are on placement in a community that has a high ethnic population, try to find out the extent of the population in the area.

Alternatively, explore for yourself the data and compare this with other census statistics to gain a sense of proportion of the numbers of immigrants, migrants and emigrants over a period of time, in order to understand the rate of changes in the UK or local neighbourhoods.

As this activity is based on your own observations, there is no outline answer at the end of the chapter.

Being sensitive to differences

There is a danger in societies that being different from the mainstream is equated with being inferior. Therefore, as Thompson (2001) points out, being sensitive to differences prevents:

- alienating people – by making groups feel that they do not belong to society;
- invalidating people – which creates the feeling that views are not valid because they are different;
- missing key issues – by not noticing crucial factors because we are not sensitive to the significance they have for others;
- becoming part of the problem – which is failing to challenge discrimination and oppression and thereby playing a part in their continuance.

Focusing on culture

Culture is a complex and multifaceted social phenomenon that affects our lives. To be an effective communicator with culturally diverse patients, a nurse has to be able to understand different social structures and norms that influence values and behaviour in different societies.. By having this knowledge, nurses can understand unfamiliar behaviour patterns and attitudes without dismissing or devaluing them. On a practical level, this requires speaking to patients in appropriate ways with knowledge of culturally congruent language to manage intercultural healthcare episodes.

Definitions relating to culture

Let's look at some common definitions. Leininger (1997, p175) defines culture as *a common collectivity of beliefs, values, shared understandings and patterns of behaviour of a designated group of people*. The term 'culture' is often used to describe a very large social group based on a shared national origin. It can also refer to a regional culture reflecting a collective sense of being through activities, traditions and language contained within a geographical area, or to an organisational culture that implies an ethical ethos or political stance.

Generally speaking, culture is a learned social experience that is often handed down through generations, thus providing a continuing connectedness with others in a community. Over periods of time, social rules and norms are established that provide a code of behaviour for the community and that also provide safety and security. Within the culture, there may be differential status roles and yet persons connected within the culture are regarded as like-minded persons, whereas someone who is not part of the culture can be treated with mistrust and suspicion.

According to Henley and Schott (1999), culture affects every aspect of daily life: how we think, feel and behave, and make decisions and judgements. Culture can be defined as 'how we do and view things in our group', which in large part is acquired unconsciously in early childhood (Hofstede, 1991).

ACTIVITY 8.4   PRACTICAL

To appreciate how culture is learned, identify and describe one family custom or tradition in your own family or community group. Ask your parent, grandparent or an elder where the custom originated. Has the custom or tradition changed over the years and can they tell you why? This might help you understand how some cultures become assimilated into the mainstream, or not, and relates to the next topics of multiculturalism and acculturation.

Can you also think of a custom that you have adopted, but that is relatively new in your family or social group? Can you trace why this has happened, and the source of this custom?

As this activity is based on your own observations, there is no outline answer at the end of the chapter.

Multiculturalism is the term used to describe a heterogeneous society in which many diverse cultural groups coexist with some general 'etic' characteristics, which are shared by the entire group, and some 'emic' perspectives, which are unique to particular groups within the larger multicultural group. Bearing in mind the discussion above on migration, which indicates a society that is progressively more mobile, society is increasingly considered to be global due to changes in demographics and an interdependent world economy. The movement towards shared cultural characteristics and social mores is due to increased interracial marriage or relationships between communities and the increased use of media and the internet to shared cultural behaviours and beliefs. Conversely, this can also create a cultural conservatism, where groups invest energy to retain cultural differences in an attempt to ward off change and a diminishing of their cultural beliefs.

Acculturation represents an adaptive cultural process whereby biological, environmental and traditional forms of culture adapt to prevailing contextual mores, in order to survive or to maintain economic and social status. This can be seen in groups who have moved from an agricultural life to an urban existence, and is particularly evident in the creation of food and eating rituals, for example a current TV cooking programme that teaches Asian women how to make club sandwiches.

A further example is family size – in many cultures a large family represents security and survival, whereas for survival in an economic and materially dependent industrial society, small families are more prevalent.

'Cultural diversity' describes the differences among cultural groups. Diversity is becoming the norm in our societies rather than the exception and covers a wide range of attributes such as nationality, ethnic origin, gender, educational background, geographic location, economic status, language, politics and religion. There can also be diversity within the same societal groups, such as age and work cultures. For example, teenagers may have a different outlook on work from generations that have experienced the financial stringencies of the post-Second World War period.

There is also a cultural diversity in health and social care settings among professions, for example physicians, social workers, healthcare assistants, nurses, administrators, porters and physiotherapists each can have their own cultural identities, rituals and practices that can affect decisions and the allocation of tasks.

'**Cultural relativism**' refers to the understanding that cultures are not inferior or superior to one another and that there is no method of measuring the value of one culture against another. Furthermore, within cultures individuals will ascribe different levels of meaning and importance to cultural beliefs and behaviours. This means that, just because an individual appears to belong to a culture, they may not follow all the practices of that culture, particularly if they have adopted elements of acculturalisation. The implications for nurses are that some may have made major modifications in their cultural beliefs to be either more extensive or more moderate. Consequently, customs, attitudes, rituals and beliefs have to be understood according to the individual needs of each patient.

The antonym to cultural relativism is 'ethnocentrism', which is where a group will believe their nation, culture or group is superior. There are several examples of this in history, for example Hitler in the last century in Europe, and more recently in the Balkans. To be proud of one's ethnicity is acceptable, but if this is taken to extremes, oppression is the outcome. **Discrimination** is another form of ethnocentrism where groups in society are marginalised, such as the physically or mentally disabled, those in poverty or homeless, and persons with HIV. When access to healthcare is inhibited or age and racial discrimination are at play, these are subtle forms of **ethnocentricity**.

Ethnicity derives from the Greek word 'ethnos' meaning 'people'. An ethnic group is a social grouping of people who share a common racial, geographical, religious or historical culture. Ethnicity is different from culture in that it represents a symbolic awareness of elements that bind people together in a social context. Ethnicity is a deliberate and chosen awareness of norms and symbols, whereas culture does not always involve a conscious awareness and commitment to a cultural identity.

ACTIVITY 8.5   PRACTICAL

The discussions above highlight the many different interpretations of culture. Take a few moments to jot down the words and phrases you can think of in response to the word 'culture'. There are no right or wrong answers to this.

- What does your list reveal to you about your attitude to culture?
- In what ways does it reflect your own cultural background?
- How can you use these notes to improve your approach to culturally congruent care?

As this activity is based on your own reflection, there is no outline answer at the end of the chapter.

Communicating with cultural diversity

Communication is often the first barrier when considering cultural diversity. The language barrier may be the most obvious difficulty to overcome, and if English is a second language, there may not be complete mastery of the terminology and ways of describing problems and symptoms. In addition, there may be conflicting assumptions and expectations about health and healthcare due to culturally based health beliefs. This is, however, the tip of the iceberg, as there are many other, not always evident, cultural barriers that lie beneath the water's surface. Figure 8.1 illustrates these factors, those that may be readily evident and those that may not be so evident in initial communications but that will have an impact on the effectiveness of communication and the relationship between patient and nurse.

Communication requires recognition of care alternatives, confidence in cross-cultural communication skills and the ability to analyse situations in specifically situated contexts. Leininger (1988) has suggested that there are three possible modes of support: *cultural preservation*, *cultural negotiation* and *cultural repatterning*.

Cultural preservation

This facilitates the retention or incorporation of helpful or harmless health- and illness-related practices, such as traditional herbal teas and ethnic foods, which are integral cultural practices. Wearing garments that are specific to a designation or talismans that maintain cultural beliefs should be retained, for the meaning and symbolism of these artefacts are important to maintaining health in many cultures. Respect for these artefacts is paramount and they should be valued as inclusive contributions to health maintenance.

Cultural negotiation, or accommodation

This means bringing together the biomedical and the cultural by negotiation and understanding. For example, in some cultures a bed facing in a certain direction can

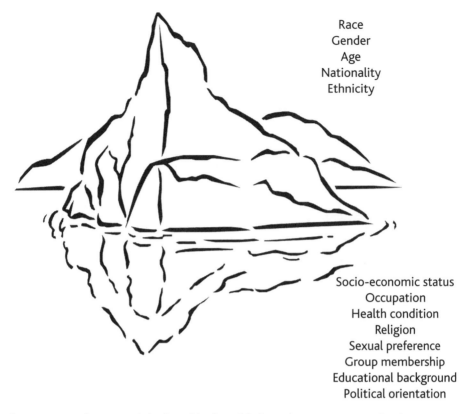

Race
Gender
Age
Nationality
Ethnicity

Socio-economic status
Occupation
Health condition
Religion
Sexual preference
Group membership
Educational background
Political orientation

Figure 8.1: Iceberg model of multicultural influences on communication.

Source: Adapted from Kreps and Kunimoto (1994).

mean the person is facing death, so turning the bed around or finding another bed facing a different direction can allay fears and improve cooperation. In another example, a family of a terminally ill child would not return the child to the unit on time for his medications. The hospital staff interpreted this as the family refusing treatment and were reluctant for the child to go on outings. On discussion, it was discovered that the family wanted to spend as much time as possible with the child because they knew he was going to die, whereas the goal of the staff was to prolong his life as much as possible by using the therapies they had devised. Negotiation between the staff and the family and exploring the conflicting goals enabled both sides to find a new understanding and a way forward, so that the staff supported the outings and the family made efforts to bring the child back on time.

Cultural repatterning, or restructuring

These are interventions that are geared to changing previously held patterns of behaviour that are having a major detrimental effect on the patient's life. In cases where there are legal consequences associated with beliefs, such as in the case of withholding permission for procedures (for example, blood transfusions, surgery or rights to die), the legal aspects of the situation have to be thoroughly considered in addition to the patient's wishes. For situations of abuse or neglect, referral should be made to specialist services for consultation and actions.

Leininger (1978) has suggested using a template of information for Culturally Diverse Clients, which could be considered as a guide for exploring individual patients' cultural needs and includes the following.

1. *Patterns or lifestyles of an individual or group.*

2. *Specific cultural values, norms, and experiences of a patient or group regarding the health and caring behaviours of their culture.*

3. *Cultural taboos or myths.*

4. *The worldview and ethnocentric tendencies of an individual (or group).*

5. *General features the patient (or group) perceives as different from, or similar to, other cultures in or near their environment.*

6. *The health and life-care rituals and rites of passage to maintain health and avoid illness.*

7. *Folk and professional health–illness systems.*

8. *Detailed caring behaviours and nursing care for self and others.*

9. *Indicators of cultural changes and acculturation processes influencing health care.*

(Leininger, 1978, pp88–9)

ACTIVITY 8.6   REFLECTIVE

Take a moment to think about your own cultural roots. Following the guide above, see if you can complete the template by describing your cultural roots. When you have done this, think of a culture that you know very little about and spend some time researching in the library or on the internet for information that would complete the template for that group. Maybe you have encountered a person from a group that you know little about and can use this as an opportunity to enhance your understanding.

Then think about how you would communicate with a person to provide you with the information if you were to do this in a practice setting. You could imagine being on a ward, in an accident and emergency department, a community health clinic, a person's home or with a homeless person on an outreach experience, or with a child or a person with mental health problems or a person with learning difficulties. Each of these situations requires an additional level of sensitivity from the nurse and adjustment, so take these into consideration.

As this activity is based on your own reflection and observations, there is no outline answer at the end of the chapter.

The skills that a nurse uses to communicate with patients cross-culturally are an extension of the skills previously discussed in this book. However, they can be embellished by the following suggested questions.

- Can you tell me something about the reasons you are seeking health care?
- Can you tell me something about how a person in your culture would be cared for if they had a similar condition?
- Have you been treated for a similar problem in the past? (If the patient answers yes, more information about the precise nature of treatment is elicited.)
- Can you tell me what people do in your culture/community to remain healthy?
- Can you tell me something about the foods you like and how they are prepared?
- Are there any special cultural beliefs about your illness that might help me give you better care?

Multicultural Britain

Britain is regarded as one of the most ethnically diverse countries in Europe (Narayanasamy and White, 2005). Therefore, healthcare providers must deliver a service that is culturally sensitive, competent and appropriate to meet specific and diverse needs (Narayanasamy, 2002). However, Narayanasamy and White (2005) argue from a historical perspective (Cortis, 1993; Wilkins, 1993) that, since its inception, the NHS can be viewed as a service that was created to meet the healthcare needs of the British people. Its provision:

evolved around British social and family patterns, embracing religious and cultural beliefs . . . It responded predominantly to the expectations and health needs of the indigenous population in 1948.

(Narayanasamy and White, 2005, p103)

THEORY SUMMARY

Ethnocentrism

The process of socialisation into the occupation of nursing carries with it the need to internalise the dominant cultural values. Because of this, nursing is not culture-free, but is embedded in cultural values that pervade all aspects of care, practice and knowledge, including CIPS. So nursing is culturally determined. If this is neither acknowledged nor understood then nurses can be charged with being guilty of gross ethnocentrism (Stokes, 1991). In the words of Parfitt:

Nurses who hold ethnocentric views will be unable to interpret their patients' behaviour appropriately as they will judge it according to the norms of their own behaviour.

(1998, p52)

The extent to which ethnocentric cultural values still prevail in the NHS is an interesting and crucial question. According to Parfitt (1998, p50), the NHS *reflects the cultural norm of not only the white majority but the middle class white majority*. From this critical position, privileged white British values and assumptions are taken as 'common sense' and 'right and proper', against which ethnic and cultural minorities are located and labelled as 'the other'. This has obvious implications for the prevalence of institutional racism and witting or unwitting prejudice among healthcare workers.

Sawley (2001) highlights racist incidents in nursing and healthcare. These include black colleagues being referred to in derogatory terms; white relatives being allowed to use the patients' toilets while Asian relatives are barred; white staff making racist remarks against Asians; and Asian patients not being permitted to have large numbers of visitors, while white patients were not subjected to such controls. These practices are clearly reflective of racist prejudice in the wider societal context, which Figure 8.2 may help illustrate.

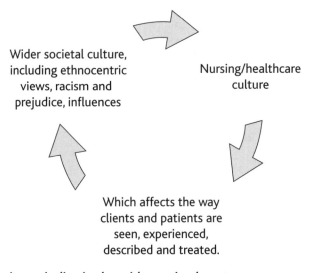

Figure 8.2: Racist prejudice in the wider societal context.

Cultural competence

Cultural competence refers to an ability to interact effectively with people of different cultures. It is is comprised of four components:

- awareness of one's own cultural world-view;
- attitude towards cultural differences;
- knowledge of different cultural practices and world-views;
- cross-cultural skills.

Developing cultural competence results in an ability to understand, communicate with, and effectively interact with people across cultures – in short, to be culturally sensitive.

Anderson et al. (2007) explored the principles of involving the community to strengthen cultural competence in nurse education, practice and research in order to reduce the health disparities in communities. The findings of these researchers included the importance of reducing and levelling differences in power between practitioners and the community. It also clearly emerged that communication and relationships between healthcare workers and community members have to be culturally appropriate and that it was crucially important to work hard to develop trust. Overall, reflecting the importance of the 'I–Thou' rather than the 'I–It' relationship discussed in Chapters 2 and 7, it was considered essential that interventions were done 'with' rather than 'to' people.

In a complementary argument, focusing on the experience of pain, Lovering (2006) asserted that patients and health professionals bring their own cultural attitudes to interpret and talk about patients' pain experience, with the health professionals' knowledge and attitudes dominating. Lovering suggested that this situation could be improved through learning about the differing cultural attitudes towards pain held by both cultural groups and health staff. The rational for this was that, through such learning, staff and patients/clients from differing cultural groups can work with each other as opposed to the former 'doing to' the latter.

Cioffi (2006) conducted qualitative research in Australia. This explored experiences of interaction between nurses and minority ethnic clients/patients. Nurses and clients/patients from Asian or Middle Eastern Islamic backgrounds were interviewed individually about perceptions of the care provided. Issues identified were tensions arising from the Islamic groups' fear of discrimination, the requirements of visiting relatives, nurses' gender, perceived cultural differences and problems of communication and information exchange.

In support of all of the above, Gerrish et al. (1996) recommended ways in which transcultural healthcare might be transmitted. According to these authors, the overarching need is the development of cultural sensitivity: in this context, the practitioner should assume the role of tourist (with the good manners that go with that role), reflexive honesty (including the ways in which power may be distributed in favour of the health practitioner), exploration of the cultural meanings of ethnicity, striving for intercultural communication, and a strong focus to eradicate all forms of racism, including institutional.

Culture without cultural awareness

In the context of ethnocentricity, culture and institutional racism, as with prejudice, the irony is that members of dominant cultures are likely to remain unaware that they have a specific culture. In terms of their social identity, as discussed above, what they regard as normal and universal assumptions, beliefs and behaviours are only 'normal' relative to their class, time and social groupings. In contrast, those who have grown up as minority ethnic group members, or who have lived outside or away from their own society, are much more likely to be acutely aware of the influence of culture by being cultural 'outsiders'.

Transcultural nursing

As was made clear in Chapter 1, 'caring' needs to be appraised through a transcultural lens (Leininger, 1997). In related terms, the quest for 'self-awareness' needs to be broadened to subjecting oneself to challenges to one's assumptions (Gerrish et al., 1996), because without the opportunities for self-awareness development in this transcultural sense, healthcare workers are likely to remain insensitive to other cultural values. This speaks to relational ethics (see Chapter 2) in that the imposition of one's own values on others can be offensive and unprofessional (Baxter, 2000; MacNaught, 1994).

In the early 1970s the second author trained as a student mental health nurse. He witnessed several examples of cultural insensitivity through British nurses renaming their ethnically different colleagues with British names. So, for example, a male colleague from the Republic of the Philippines, whose first name was difficult to pronounce by British colleagues, became 'Fred'. Less understandably, a Danish nurse named 'Elsa' was renamed 'Elsie'.

Fortunately, cultural sensitivity seems to be beginning to impact nursing more now. For example, Narayanasamy and White (2005) argue that healthcare services should be culturally responsive and that the cultural healthcare needs of ethnic minority groups are still not adequately met. Specifically, there is a failure of multicultural education, structures and policies, and transcultural healthcare practice (Gerrish et al., 1996), which may be being met, at least in part, by developing models of transcultural nursing.

THE ACCESS MODEL OF TRANSCULTURAL NURSING (NARAYANASAMY, 2002)

Assessment:	The assessment process focuses on the cultural dimensions of the client's lifestyle, and beliefs and practices about health.
Communication:	The nurse strives for awareness of, and differences in, variations in verbal and non-verbal responses.
Cultural negotiation and compromise:	The nurse strives to become aware of aspects of other people's cultures, understand their viewpoints, and tries to explain their problems in an acceptable and accessible way.
Establishing respect and rapport:	What is required is a therapeutic relationship which embodies genuine respect for varieties in culture beliefs and values.
Sensitivity:	Nurses deliver diverse culturally sensitive care to diverse cultural groups.
Safety:	Clients/patients are enabled to derive a sense of cultural safety (see introduction to this chapter).

Transcultural care

Robb and Douglas (2004) also addressed social identities – memberships of particular groups said to share common experiences and needs. These are characterised by ethnicity, gender, disability, age and sexuality, all of which structure people's everyday experiences, including being in receipt of healthcare. These can be used to define people as 'other' or 'different', against a supposed 'norm'.

ACTIVITY 8.7   PRACTICAL

A Bangladeshi woman is admitted to hospital for two weeks to undergo an operation. Afterwards, she reports that, while in hospital, she felt stupid because of her lack of English. 'Two nurses neglected me. I'm not sure if it was because of the colour of my skin or because of a language barrier. I'm still not sure what operation I had, and why.'

In small groups, discuss:

- What is the nature of the communication problem experienced by the woman?
- Whose problem is it?
- What are the consequences for the speaker?

As this activity is based on your own observations, there is no outline answer at the end of the chapter.

The questions raised in Activity 8.7 hopefully demonstrate the complexities of the issues, rather than easy answers. The answers you came up with will relate to your understanding of the nature of 'difference', how it is produced and how it should be responded to. For example, one possible answer is that the 'cause' of the problem was the woman's poor command of spoken English coupled with her lack of confidence, either because of her language difficulties or her cultural background.

However, equally, it could be argued that the communication problem arose because of the hospital's failure to address indirect and direct discrimination in its practices. Indirect discrimination was apparent in the failure to take account of the diverse needs of patients by, for example, failing to ensure the provision of bilingual workers or interpreters available for the main community languages in the area. Direct discrimination was apparent in how the two nurses ignored the woman.

The point is that nurses, like all humans, understand 'difference' differently. Related to social cognition-based discussions in this book on labelling, 'cognitive miserliness' (see Chapter 4) and prejudices, health workers often associate 'difference' with the membership of particular groups. These groups are seen to have specific qualities, ways of communicating and communication needs, such as those described in Activity 8.8 below:

ACTIVITY 8.8 PRACTICAL

Consider the following statements, and rate them on the following scale:

0	2	4	6	8
absolutely untrue	probably untrue	not sure	probably true	absolutely true

- Latin people use their bodies and hands more expressively than British people when they are communicating.
- Asian women lack confidence in talking with white nurses.
- People with learning disabilities find speaking in groups very stressful.
- Women let their emotions get the better of them when they're under pressure.
- The Scots and the Irish are always looking for a fight rather than trying to resolve differences of opinion through discussion.
- Lesbians don't like being cared for by male nurses.

Share your results with other people in your group and discuss.

As this activity is based on your own observations, there is no outline answer at the end of the chapter.

Focusing on diversity

Diversity is about us as individual beings. However, as we have discussed earlier, society is made up of a variety of groups and we will explore those groups in this section from a sociological perspective. Again, it is these differences that will influence the character and nature of our interpersonal interactions with patients and fellow workers. We will explore socio-economic position, race and culture, gender, sexual orientation, age and disability.

Socio-economic position

This is also described as a person's class and is closely linked to factors such as income, wealth and social status. The ONS uses a classification system to gather data on the population that is constructed around employment roles and economic output. The first detailed classification was designed in 1928 and was intended to identify differences in economic distribution and status.

SOCIAL CLASS BASED ON OCCUPATION

I   Professional etc. occupations

II Managerial and technical occupations

III   Skilled occupations
  (N)   non-manual
  (M)   manual
IV   Partly skilled occupations
V   Unskilled occupations

The occupation groups included in each of these categories were selected in such a way as to bring together, as far as possible, people with similar levels of occupational skill. In general, each occupation group was assigned as a whole to one or other social class and no account was taken of differences between individuals in the same occupation group, for example differences in education. However, for persons having the employment status of foreman or manager, the following additional rules applied:

  (a)   each occupation was given a basic social class;

  (b)   persons of foreman status whose basic social class was IV or V were allocated to Social Class III;

  (c)   persons of manager status were allocated to Social Class II with certain exceptions.

(Adapted from Rose and Pevalin, 2005, p5)

This ethos has prevailed and a further more comprehensive classification system was developed in 1951.

SOCIO-ECONOMIC GROUPS

Classification by Socio-economic Group (SEG) was introduced in 1951 and extensively amended in 1961. The classification aimed to bring together people with jobs of similar social and economic status. The allocation of occupied persons to SEG was determined by considering their employment status and occupation (and industry, though for practical purposes no direct reference was made since it was possible in Great Britain to use classification by occupation as a means of distinguishing effectively those engaged in agriculture).

  1.1   Employers in industry, commerce, etc. (large establishments)
  1.2   Managers in central and local government, industry, commerce, etc. (large establishments)
  2.1   Employers in industry, commerce, etc. (small establishments)
  3.   Professional workers – self-employed
  4.   Professional workers – employees

5.1 Intermediate non-manual workers – ancillary workers and artists

5.2 Intermediate non-manual workers – foremen and supervisors non-manual

6. Junior non-manual workers

7. Personal service workers

8. Foremen and supervisors – manual

9. Skilled manual workers

10. Semi-skilled manual workers

11. Unskilled manual workers

12. Own-account workers (other than professional)

13. Farmers – employers and managers

14. Farmers – own account

15. Agricultural workers

16. Members of armed forces

17. Inadequately described and not stated occupations

(Adapted from Rose and Pevalin, 2005, p7)

However, this has been subject to criticism as being inadequately sensitive for contemporary statistical analysis and for capturing the inadequacies of the state in providing equal access to health, education, housing and employment, so a further classification model has been developed.

OPERATIONAL CATEGORIES OF THE NATIONAL STATISTICS SOCIO-ECONOMIC CLASSIFICATION (NS-SEC)

L1 Employers in Large Establishments
L2 Higher Managerial Occupations
L3 Higher Professional Occupations
    L3.1 'Traditional' employees
    L3.2 'New' employees
    L3.3 'Traditional' self-employed
    L3.4 'New' self-employed
L4 Lower Professional and Higher Technical Occupations
    L4.1 'Traditional' employees
    L4.2 'New' employees
    L4.3 'Traditional' self-employed
    L4.4 'New' self-employed
L5 Lower Managerial Occupations
L6 Higher Supervisory Occupations
L7 Intermediate Occupations
    L7.1 Intermediate clerical and administrative occupations

L7.2   Intermediate service occupations
L7.3   Intermediate technical and auxiliary occupations
L7.4   Intermediate engineering occupations
L8   Employers in Small Organisations
L8.1   Employers in small organisations in industry, commerce, services, etc.
L8.2   Employers in small organisations in agriculture
L9   Own-account Workers
L9.1   Own-account workers (non-professional)
L9.2   Own-account workers in agriculture
L10   Lower Supervisory Occupations
L11   Lower Technical Occupations
L11.1   Lower technical craft occupations
L11.2   Lower technical process operative occupations
L12   Semi-routine Occupations
L12.1   Semi-routine sales occupations
L12.2   Semi-routine service occupations
L12.3   Semi-routine technical occupations
L12.4   Semi-routine operative occupations
L12.5   Semi-routine agricultural occupations
L12.6   Semi-routine clerical occupations
L12.7   Semi-routine childcare occupations
L13   Routine Occupations
L13.1   Routine sales and service occupations
L13.2   Routine production occupations
L13.3   Routine technical occupations
L13.4   Routine operative occupations
L13.5   Routine agricultural occupations
L14   Never Worked and Long-term Unemployed
L14.2   Long-term unemployed
L15   Full-time Students
L16   Occupations not stated or inadequately described
L17   Not classifiable for other reasons

(Adapted from Rose and Pevalin, 2005, p17)

The historical development of these classification systems indicates the increasing complexity of the structure of our society. For a full discussion and report on the current classification system used by the ONS, see Rose and Pevalin (2005).

Politically and sociologically, class differentials have been the subject of much debate and continue to be used to delineate social divisions in society and the distribution of wealth. The impact of social origins on life chances continues to be researched (Platt, 2005). The gap in the share of income between the richest and the poorest has increased and also employment and educational achievements continue to be determined by social background (Devine et al., 2004). Added to this are economic changes that are affecting society, such as the decrease in traditional working-class employment in the manufacturing industry and the increase in the service industry.

The development of the welfare state in the twentieth century is held to be responsible for a broader middle-class grouping and the emergence of other categories, such as gender and ethnicity, that are competing with class distinctions as having an effect on life's chances.

The implication for nursing is that we are expected to work with persons from all aspects of life and, when communicating with persons from different socio-economic backgrounds, it is important not to make assumptions based upon class stereotypes. People move from one group to another and can be affected by a variety of circumstances. There is a danger that collusion can occur between similar groups and issues overlooked, for example middle-class health visitors overlooking child abuse in middle-class families. The use of restricted language should not be confused with levels of comprehension. Each patient is entitled to full explanations of their treatments and interventions in a manner that is helpful and neutral from assumptions, for example that the most educated do not need explanations and those with less education need more. It is the clarity and quality of the explanation that is relevant and everyone needs reassurance regardless of their socio-economic position.

Race and culture

The UK has a population that is composed of a wide variety of cultures, religions and languages. There are over 100 different languages spoken in London schools. While there are differing concentrations of multiculturalism throughout the four countries, the UK is no longer a white homogeneous nation. To think so is to devalue the minority cultures within our society and disregard aspects of people's lives. This denial can lead to racist attitudes and can act as a barrier to good practice in healthcare. Communication and interpersonal interactions need to be ethnically sensitive and anti-racist. Assumptions, for example on skin colour determining biological differences, have the potential to be used as arguments for the destructive mythology of racial inferiority. Taking the time to understand cultural and ethnic beliefs and practices is needed, as well as listening to the stories of friends and colleagues who have been harassed or abused through racism – if they trust you enough to share their stories.

Gender

In most societies, there are recognisable differences between men and women and a male/female divide that has various codes and expectations of behaviour and responses in social interaction. By the age of two, infants can recognise the differences through hair and clothes, aided by significant gender stereotyping that is prevalent in most societies. The extent to which gender differences are innate or learned is, though, the subject of debate. Social constructionists claim that gender is constructed through everyday discourse and reinforced through communication patterns, whereas evolutionary theorists argue that gender variations in behaviour arise only from biological differences. The jury is still out, but there seems a strong case for both nature and nurture to play a role in varying degrees.

Studies of gender-related communication behaviours suggest that women prefer less interpersonal space, touch and are touched more, gesture less, look and are looked at more and smile more frequently. Social skills inventories have revealed consistent gender differences on various dimensions, females scoring higher on measures of emotional expressivity and sensitivity (see Hargie, 2006). Males prefer to be more directive, self-opinioned and explicit, whereas females tend to be more indirect, use a greater number of uncertainties (it could be) (might be), that is, passive speech styles, speak for longer periods and refer more to emotions. There are inconsistencies in the studies reporting these behaviours and the general view is that gender is something we 'do' rather than something we 'are'.

The development of feminism and the critical feminist movement has helped to widen our understanding of women's place in society and the contribution they make. There remain concerns over the unequal distribution of power and life chances between men and women. To overcome these concerns there continues to be a need to retain a critical view of how women are treated in healthcare settings to ensure that their needs are not overlooked and that male dominance is not reinforced or legitimised. It is important to ensure that women's problems are constructed in women's terms and not men's, and that stereotypical gender expectations are challenged if they are without evidence or foundation. There are specific examples of female-related health problems (for example, sexual abuse and depression) that may pass unnoticed unless highlighted.

Men can also experience problems associated with sexism when rigid stereotyping expects certain responses from men on how they are expected to think, feel and act. This is particularly evident at times of bereavement.

When men and women interact within a context of gender inequality, barriers to communication and interpersonal relationships can inhibit effective assessment and health interventions. The danger is that gender inequality can exacerbate or reinforce existing problems (for example, low self-esteem) and lack of opportunity to speak, describe or express ideas on problems that are being presented. The prevailing advice is to assume a neutral communication style and be aware of using your own gender stereotypical behaviour in interactions.

Sexual orientation

Taking the biological view that sexuality is purely, or primarily, a biological phenomenon, and heterosexuality deemed to be natural and normal, inevitably defines homosexuality as unnatural and abnormal. This view, however, rules out those in society who have chosen an alternative sexual orientation. The social and psychological dimensions of sexuality are relevant in this discussion as they provide explanations for an alternative view of sexuality that cannot be ignored or marginalised. If not considered, the only concept of sexuality is one that is limited to the biological argument and has the potential to lead to misunderstandings, prejudice and discrimination.

It has to be acknowledged that gay and lesbian relationships, which are accepted in some cultures, are not in others. In many countries, same-sex couples could face severe punishment or death, whereas in other countries they can be recognised legally. This creates an additional dilemma for the health professional who, on the one hand, is prepared to help persons regardless of their sexual orientation, but who, on the other hand, will also take into account the beliefs of persons in their care that may not, through reasons of faith or culture, accept homosexuality. Nurses may also have their own cultural beliefs, which could be challenged by this situation. As with other diverse groups under discussion, respect, fairness and dignity are important features of working in a professional and non-judgemental manner and are the precepts to be guided by in these encounters in the healthcare context.

Age

Ageism is a term generally applied to discrimination against older persons, although it can be applied to children. When applied to older persons it can be characterised by a number of factors.

- Marginalisation – older people and their needs are rarely seen as a priority or a central concern.
- Dehumanisation – older people are represented as 'over the hill' and of little use to society.
- Infantalisation – older people tend to be treated like children, for example by using first names without asking the person if this is acceptable.

The phenomena of social ageing, or how we behave in social encounters towards each other, and our understanding of the differences between ourselves and others as we age or change are thought to be achieved through communication. Our own age, and the age of those with whom we interact, shape our responses, behaviours and expectations. Therefore, we take the target of our responses into consideration and frame them accordingly. So, for example, a reward for a child would be 'you're a clever little person', for an adolescent 'you have really grown up' and for an older person it could be 'I find your ideas very interesting'. Adapting to make the apposite response is how we reduce ageism and at the same time guard against being patronising.

Reaction times, speech recognition and the capacity for information processing slows down with ageing; however, this happens at a different rate for different individuals. Older people have often had years of experience in dealing with people from different backgrounds and in different situations, and have gained a wealth of language to use in these contexts. Regrettably, there is negative stereotyping for the older person that is transformed into the use of secondary baby talk, elderspeak and patronising talk. This is often the result of intentions to be helpful, such as slowing down or simplification of messages and clarification exercises, for example raising the volume of the voice, deliberate articulation and diminutives such as 'dear' or 'love'. These patterns, as well as being demeaning, have a negative effect on the self-identity of elderly persons and reinforce their sense of loss of control and dependency.

The implications for the nurse are to consider pitching responses at the apposite level, having first assessed the ability (rather than chronological age) of the other person. There is also a danger of concentrating on the physical needs of the older person and not considering their rights or choices.

Disability

Disability is often viewed as a physical problem that stands in the way of normal social functioning. An alternative view is that social attitudes to disability are the disabling function rather than the impairment itself. An example of this is that it is not the use of a wheelchair that bars access to buildings, it is the lack of disabled access and a ramp that causes the disability. The social model of disability draws attention to the tendency of disabled people to be marginalised, dehumanised and patronised (there are similarities here to ageism). There is a focus on limitations rather than potential and capability. There is also a lack of awareness of the barriers, both physical and attitudinal, that prevent disabled persons from becoming integrated into society. Finally, there is a tendency to focus on dependency rather than empowerment (Oliver, 1990).

Here are some suggestions for interpersonal communication concerning disabilities (adapted from DeVito, 2007).

- Avoid negative terms and terms that define the person as disabled, such as 'the disabled man' or 'the handicapped child'.

- Instead, say 'person with a disability', always emphasising the person rather than the disability. Avoid describing the person with a disability as 'abnormal'; when you define people without disabilities as 'normal', you say, in effect, that the person with the disability isn't normal.

- Treat assistive devices such as wheelchairs, canes, walkers or crutches as the personal property of the user. Don't move these out of your way; they're for the convenience of the person with the disability. Avoid leaning on a person's wheelchair – it is similar to leaning on the person.

- Shake hands with the person with the disability if you shake hands with others in the group. Don't avoid shaking hands because the individual's hand is disfigured or misshapen, for example.

- Avoid talking about the person with a disability in the third person. For example, avoid saying 'Doesn't he get around beautifully with the new crutches'. Direct your comments to the individual.

- Don't assume that people who have a disability are intellectually impaired. Slurred speech, such as may occur with cerebral palsy or cleft palate, should never be taken as indicating a low-level intellect. So be especially careful not to talk down to people, as many do.

- When you're not sure of how to act, ask. For example, if you're not sure if you should offer walking assistance, say 'Would you like me to help you into the dining room.' And, more importantly, accept the person's response. If he or she says no, then that means no! So don't insist.

- Maintain similar eye level. If the person is in a wheelchair, for example, it might be helpful for you to sit down or kneel down to maintain the same eye level.

Ethical and moral dimensions

Because there are consequences of communication and personal interactions, whether deliberate or unintentional, there are also ethical considerations to take into account. Each communication situation has a moral dimension of rightness and wrongness, where the expectation is that communication will be honest, decent, just and appropriate. These moral principles are often expected and implicit in interactions. There is an expectation that nurses will respect individuals and act within the NMC *Code of Professional Conduct* (2004b), which embodies these principles. Within a cultural context, these have to be considered and interpreted according to the respective value systems of each culture. An example is the close physical proximity in which much nursing takes place, which creates an additional layer of ethical complexity, related to intimacy, as discussed previously in Chapter 3. There are many occasions when decisions and choices about healthcare treatments and therapies have to be guided by ethical considerations, as well as concerns about the effectiveness of a chosen path and the satisfaction this will give to the patients and carers.

A first step to making decisions that take account of cultural variability is to understand the way in which culture influences how health and illness are understood by the members of a cultural group or community sharing the same values. The cultural interpretation of health and illness is based upon values and perceptions that are the product of the combination of traditions, lived experiences and the knowledge sanctioned by a particular culture. The values are often derived from the notion of health as a resource – how this features in daily lives and how this affects the productivity, effectiveness, significance and status of a person in their community.

The dominant framework for understanding the cause and treatment of ill health in the Western world is the **biomedical model**. The conceptual framework for the biomedical model is that illness is caused by the malfunctioning of a specific bodily part and the part in question needs to be treated so that the illness may be removed. The emphasis is on cure, often technical and/or pharmacological, which is based upon the broader scientific notions of control through empirical observation and driven by evidence from controlled experiments or studies. The assumption is that the model provides a truthful account of reality when compared to more primitive forms of healing and curing practices, which are not empirically based and hence irrational. The model has relevance in delivering effective solutions in certain instances; however, it is not culturally sensitive.

CASE STUDY

Alisha is 42 years old and works as a cleaner in an office building in a large UK city. She came to the UK from West Bengal, India, 22 years ago as a young bride. She barely makes a living and depends upon her work to supplement her husband's wages and support her family of five children, two of whom are adults but unemployed and living at home. In discussing her health, Alisha reveals a complex interaction of responses. If she considers the illness to be very serious she will go to the local hospital, even though she knows she will have to wait a long time to be seen and it will be difficult to explain to the nurses and doctors why she is there, because her English is limited. This is the last resort. For persistent fevers in her children she will go to the local allopathic doctor (using remedies whose effects differ from those produced by the disease), even though there will be high fees to pay, because she will not have to wait. In other instances, she may visit the homeopathic doctor, who is more affordable. She will also visit the kobiraj (the Ayurvedic practitioner). Finally, while Alisha knows that allopathic medicine will offer relief, she knows it will not cure. For this to happen, Alisha believes the underlying causes have to be dealt with and these are connected to divine forces. To solve this problem, Alisha makes offerings at the temple of the goddess Kali so that she will be appeased.

This case study gives an example of the centrality of culture in the perception of health and illness. It also illuminates the different resources and organisational structures that individuals may resort to for solutions to health problems. The notion of a divine origin of health, and models other than the biomedical utilised by Alisha to understand the cause and cure of illness, indicate a complex terrain of a cultural space where health and illness are negotiated.

ACTIVITY 8.9   REFLECTIVE

Which model of health do you think is the most effective and how will you discuss this, hypothetically, with Alisha? What are the ethical factors at play in this discussion? What other factors might you take into consideration in this discussion, for example family networks, finances and status?

Now compare this case study with the one that follows.

As this activity is based on your own reflection, there is no outline answer at the end of the chapter.

CASE STUDY

Jane, a single woman, was diagnosed with breast cancer at the age of 43. Even though Jane, who works as a hospital secretary, had good relationships with medical and nursing staff and had faith in their abilities, she decided to explore other treatment options. She surfed the internet for articles and gathered feedback from her friends and family. The most common response she found was, 'have it removed'. She thought this was good advice and made an appointment for surgery. As the date approached, she became more and more unsure. She read more articles that questioned the efficacy of surgery and she found alternative suggestions. These ranged from yoga to meditation and guided imagery. She was thinking of delaying the surgery and her friends advised her that she was losing precious time, yet she felt that the alternative approaches had more meaning for her.

ACTIVITY **8.10**   PRACTICAL

List the differences and similarities between the two cases above. What is the prevailing similarity and the most significant difference and can these be reconciled in the healthcare system we have in the UK? Can you describe the cultural origins of these two cases without stereotyping? (Hint: only use the facts that are before you.)

What can be learned from the second case and the health decisions and choices Jane has to make when she navigates the healthcare system? If you were Jane's friend, how would you advise her? Would this be different from the advice you would give as a professional? What are the moral obligations you have as a professional? (Hint: think of evidenced-based practice and your role as an advocate.)

As this activity is based on your own reflection, there is no outline answer at the end of the chapter.

Alisha's story involves shifting from one form of treatment to another depending on the nature of the illness, the location of the person in the family structure, the price and the time it takes to receive treatment and transport. These options are interwoven into a complex web of meaning involving hierarchies and resources. The treatments lie outside the biomedical model as well as engage with it, indicating a crossroads between a culture-centred approach and a biomedical approach. Here is a nexus for ethical decision making using communication skills that enable a deeper understanding of cultural values and issues.

CHAPTER SUMMARY

In this chapter we have considered the extent to which our population is changing and the need for increased understanding and awareness of multicultural needs in healthcare. We have also explored the definitions of culture and have discussed the socio-economic factors impacting today's healthcare recipients. As well as considering the diverse population needs of groups in society in relation to socio-economic position, race and culture, gender, sexual orientation, age and disability, we have examined the ethical and moral dimensions of communication and interpersonal relationships in a culturally diverse world.

KNOWLEDGE REVIEW

Having completed the chapter, how would you now rate your knowledge of the following topics?

	Good	Adequate	Poor
1. Population diversity in the UK.			
2. Ethical and moral issues concerning cultural variability.			
3. The communication needs of older people and those with disabilities.			

Where you're not confident in your knowledge of a topic, what will you do next?

Further reading

Dutte, MJ (2008) *Communicating Health: A culture-centred approach*. Cambridge: Polity Press.

Useful websites

www.ons.gov.uk/census/index.html This website has information on the National Census.

www.statistics.gov.uk/methods_quality/ns_sec/downloads/NS-SEC_Origins.pdf

www.statistics.gov.uk/pdfdir/intmigrat1106.pdf

The above two websites have information on immigration and migration.

www.womenshealthresearch.org The website for the Society for Women's Health Research.

biomedical model   a model employing the principles of biology, biochemistry, physiology and other basic sciences to solve problems in clinical medicine

blip culture   refers to contemporary healthcare cultures where there is only time for brief interpersonal exchanges between nurses and their clients/patients

communication   refers to the reciprocal and effective process in which messages are sent and received between two or more people

control   is central to good mental health; people who function well at the level of their mental health experience high levels of subjective control; the opposite is true for those who experience mental health difficulties

counterculture   refers to the consciously held negative views of a minority of individuals against the dominant culture

cultural relativism   relates to a culture or civilisation where there is the belief that concepts such as right and wrong, goodness and badness, or truth and falsehood are not absolute but change from culture to culture and situation to situation

culture   refers to the dominant mores, habits and beliefs of a group of people, usually united by their ethnic, social, sexual or other orientation

discrimination   refers to the conscious or unconscious negative views of individuals, on the basis of their ethnicity, sexual orientation or lifestyle

empathy   the ability to be attuned, and respond appropriately, to the inner experience and distress of patients and clients

ethnicity   ethnic affiliation or distinctiveness

ethnocentrism   a belief in, or assumption of, the superiority of the social or cultural group that a person belongs to

ethnocentricity   refers to the 'taken for granted' views held by members of a society, which, they believe, apply globally

eudaemonistic   basing moral value on the likelihood of actions producing happiness

evidence-based practice   refers to the combination of the best available scientific evidence and theories informing safe and effective interpersonal communication in nursing

existential-phenomenological   relating to personal experience and responsibility of the individual who is seen as a free agent and the doctrine that all knowledge comes from perceptions of what is sensed by the individual

experiential learning   learning that is derived from or relating to experience, as opposed to other methods of acquiring knowledge

Gestalt   a set of things, such as a person's thoughts and experiences, considered as a whole and regarded as amounting to more than the sum of its parts; a set of items or things that are regarded as a whole

healthy relating   refers to the use of good CIPS between nurses, their colleagues, and their patients/clients; good communication is respectful, non-exploitative, non-judgemental and formal rather than casual

humanistic   humanistic psychology implies that individuals can solve their own problems independent of cultural and organisational constraints

immigration   coming to a foreign country to settle there

individualism   from an 'individualistic' perspective, individuals are assumed to have the power to find their own solutions to their problems, independent of cultural or organisational constraining factors

interpersonal skills   are exhibited when nurses demonstrate their abilities to use evidence-based, and theory-based, styles of communication with their patients/clients and colleagues

level descriptors   a range of relative scales or values that are used to categorise, describe and sort ideas, activities or responsibilities

loss   is a feature of the subjective experience of depression or low mood

metacognitive   refers to the idea of 'thinking about thinking'; this means, in practice, thinking about the ways in which you, as a nurse, and your patients/clients, think about the ways in which you and they think

migration   going from one place to another

moral practice   in nursing refers to the respectful treatment of a patient/client as a fully human being, rather than an object or an 'it'

nurse-focused   refers to the defensive ways in which nurses often communicate with their patients/clients; these forms of communication are often guarded, withdrawn and distancing, leaving patients/clients feeling more anxious and lonely than they otherwise might be

prejudice   bigoted views held by members of one culture against members of another

professional friend   a relationship that conforms to the standards of skill, competence or character normally expected of a properly qualified and experienced person in a work environment and combines this with elements of friendship characterised by mutual assistance, approval and support

professional relationship   the connection between two or more people or groups and their involvement with one another, especially with regard to the way they behave towards and feel about one another, which is focused around an occupation as a paid job rather than as a hobby

rationalisation   finding reasons to explain or justify one's actions

reflective writing   writing that is characteristic of and expresses contemplative, analytical and careful thoughts

Rogerian principles   refers to the position that the 'core conditions' of Rogerian-informed interpersonal communication are both necessary and sufficient; these conditions are 'non-judgementalism', 'unconditional positive regard' and 'genuineness'

schemas   psychological templates, or mental structures, that we all develop to make sense of the world; they help us develop general expectations about ourselves, others, social roles and events, and how to behave in specific situations

self-awareness   our knowledge about ourselves, our motivations, and how these translate into our behaviours

self-esteem   an individual's subjective experience of the overall effectiveness they possess in the conduct of their lives; low self-esteem, therefore, indicates a lowered experience of such effectiveness

social relationship   the connection between two or more people or groups and their involvement with one another, especially with regard to the way they behave towards and feel about one another, focused around human society and how it is organised

social rules   authoritative principles set forth to guide behaviour or action that relate to the connection between two or more people or groups and their involvement with one another, especially with regard to the way they behave towards and feel about one another

social thinking   use of the mind to form thoughts, opinions, judgements and conclusions about the way in which people in groups behave and interact

suffering   individuals who are suffering exhibit high levels of distress in relation to their physical or mental anguish

theory of mind   the ways in which all human beings make inferences and guesses about what they think is going through the minds of others and what informs their behaviour

therapeutic relationship   relating to or involving activities carried out to maintain or improve somebody's health within the professional relationship defined above

transcultural   refers to a sophisticated awareness of the beliefs, feelings and behaviours of members of cultures other than one's own

unhealthy relating   an abandonment of the moral, psychological and empathic basis for caring, interpersonal communication; organisational environments will contribute to the shaping of healthy and unhealthy relating between nurses and patients/clients

References

Anderson, N, Calvillo, ER and Fongwa, MN (2007) Community-based approaches to strengthen cultural competency in nursing education. *Journal of Transcultural Nursing*, 18: 49–59.

Armstrong, AE (2006) Towards a strong virtue ethics for nursing practice. *Nursing Philosophy*, 7: 110–24.

Arnold, E. and Boggs, KU (2006) *Interpersonal Relationships: Professional communication skills for nurses*. London: Elsevier.

Arnold, E. and Boggs, KU (2007) *Interpersonal Relationships: Professional communication skills for nurses*, 5th edition. Philadelphia, PA: WB Saunders.

Augoustinos, M, Walker, I and Donaghue, N (2006) *Social Cognition: An integrated introduction*. London: Sage Publications.

Bach, S (2004) *Psychological Care in Community Nursing: A phenomenological investigation*. Ph.D. thesis, University of Manchester.

Balzer-Riley, J (2004) *Communication in Nursing*. Mosby, MO: Mosby/Elsevier.

Banister, P and Kagan, C (1985) The need for research into interpersonal skills, in Kagan, C (ed.) *Interpersonal Skills in Nursing: Research and applications*. London: Croom Helm, pp44–60.

Baron-Cohen, S (2003) *The Essential Difference: Men, women and the extreme male brain*. London: Basic Books.

Bateson, G (1979) *Mind and Nature*. New York: Dutton.

Baxter, C (2000) Antiracist practice: achieving competency and maintaining professional standards, in Thompson, T and Mathias, P (eds) *Lyttle's Mental Health and Disorder*. Edinburgh: Bailliere Tindall.

Beck, AT, Rush, AJ, Shaw, BF and Emery, G (1979) *Cognitive Therapy of Depression*. New York: Guilford.

Bendall, E (1976) Learning for reality. *Journal of Advanced Nursing*, 1: 3–9.

Bendall, E (2006) 30th Anniversary commentary on Bendall E. 1976 'Learning for reality'. *Journal of Advanced Nursing*, 30th Anniversary Issue.

Benner, P and Wrubel, J (1988) The primacy of caring. *American Journal of Nursing*, 88(8): 1073–5.

Benner, P, Tanner, C and Chesla, C (1996) *Expertise in Nursing Practice: Caring, clinical judgement, and ethics*. New York: Springer.

Bowlby, J (1988) *A Secure Base: Clinical applications of attachment theory*. London: Routledge.

Broadbent, M, Jarman, H and Berk, M (2002) Improving competence in emergency mental health triage. *Accident & Emergency Nursing*, 10: 155–62.

Brown, B, Crawford, P and Carter, R (2006) *Evidence-based Health Communication*. Maidenhead: Open University Press and McGraw-Hill Education.

Brykczynska, G (1997) A brief overview of the epistemology of caring, in Brykczynska, G (ed.) *Caring: The compassion and wisdom of nursing*, London: Arnold/Allen Lane, pp1–9.

Buber, M (1958) *I and Thou*, 2nd edition. New York: Charles Scribner's Sons.

Burnard, P (1996) *Acquiring Interpersonal Skills: A handbook of experiential learning for health professionals*, 2nd edition. London: Chapman and Hall.

Burnard, P (2003) Ordinary chat and therapeutic conversation: phatic communication and mental health nursing. *Journal of Psychiatric and Mental Health Nursing*, 10(6): 678–82.

Caris-Verhallen, WM, Kerkstra, A and Bensing, JM (1999) Non-verbal behaviour in nurse–elderly patient communication. *Journal of Advanced Nursing*, 29: 808–18.

Chant, S, Jenkinson, T, Randle, J and Russell, G (2002) Communication skills: some problems in nursing education and practice. *Journal of Clinical Nursing*, 11: 12–21.

Charlton, CR, Dearing, KS, Berry, JA and Johnson, MJ (2008) Nurse practitioners' communication styles and their impact on patient outcomes: an integrated literature review. *Journal of the American Academy of Nurse Practitioners*, 20: 382–8.

Cioffi, J (2006) Culturally diverse patient–nurse interactions on acute care wards. *International Journal of Nursing Practice*, 12(6): 319–25.

Clarke, JB and Wheeler, SJ (1992) A view of the phenomenon of caring in nursing practice. *Journal of Advanced Nursing*, 17: 1283–90.

Clay, M and Povey, R (1983) Moral reasoning and the student nurse. *Journal of Advanced Nursing*, 8: 297–302.

Coffield, F, Moseley, D, Hall, E and Ecclestone, K (2004) *Learning Styles and Pedagogy in Post-16 Learning: A systematic and critical review.* London: Learning and Skills Research Centre.

Cortis, JD (1993) Transcultural nursing: appropriateness for Britain. *Journal of Advances in Health and Nursing Care*, 12(4): 67–77.

Dai, DY and Sternberg, RJ (eds) (2004) *Motivation, Emotion and Cognition*. Mahwah, NJ: Lawrence Erlbaum.

Davidson, C (1985) The theoretical antecedents to interpersonal skills training, in Kagan, C (ed.) *Interpersonal Skills in Nursing: Research and applications*. London: Croom Helm, pp22–43.

Department of Health (DH) (2001) *Working Together – Learning Together: A framework for lifelong learning for the NHS*. London: Department of Health.

Department of Health (DH) (2004) *Getting Over the Wall: How the NHS is improving the patient's experience*. London: Department of Health.

Department of Health (DH) (2006) *The Expert Patients Programme*. Available online at www.dh.gov.uk (accessed 19 June 2009).

Devine, F, Savage, M, Crompton, R and Scott, J (eds) (2004) *Rethinking Class: Identities, Cultures and Lifestyles*. Basingstoke: Palgrave.

DeVito, JA (2007) *The Interpersonal Communication Book*, 11th edition. London: Pearson Education.

Duncan-Grant, A (2001) *Clinical Supervision Activity among Mental Health Nurses: A critical organizational ethnography*. Portsmouth: Nursing Praxis International.

Edelman, RJ (2000) *The Psychosocial Aspects of the Health Care Process.* Harlow: Prentice Hall.

Egan, EG (1998) *The Skilled Helper: A problem management approach to helping*, 6th edition. Pacific Grove, CA: Brooks Cole.

European Union (EU) (2004) *Enabling Good Health for All: A reflection process for a new EU strategy*. Available online at http://ec.europa.eu/health/ph_overview/ Documents/byrne_reflection_en.pdf (accessed 19 June 2009).

Fennell, M (1999) *Overcoming Low Self-esteem: A self-help guide using cognitive behavioural techniques.* London: Robinson.

Fiske, ST and Taylor, SE (1991) *Social Cognition*, 2nd edition. New York: McGraw-Hill.

Frost, PJ, Dutton, JE, Worlen, MC and Wilson, A (2000) Narratives of compassion in organizations, in Fineman, S (ed.) *Emotion in Organizations*, 2nd edition. London: Sage Publications.

Gerrish, K, Husband, C and Mackenzie, J (1996) *Nursing for a Multi-ethnic Society.* Buckingham: Open University Press.

Gilbert, P and Leahy, R (eds) (2007) *The Therapeutic Relationship in the Cognitive Behavioural Psychotherapies.* Hove: Routledge.

Goffman, E (1972) *Strategic Interaction.* New York: Ballantine.

Goleman, D (2006) *Social Intelligence: The new science of human relationships.* London: Hutchinson.

Gosling, D and Moon, J (2001) *How To Use Learning Outcomes and Assessment Criteria.* London: SEEC.

Grant, A (2002) Tales from the order of received wisdom (or some contemporary problems with mental health nurse education in Britain). *Journal of Psychiatric and Mental Health Nursing*, 9: 622–7.

Grant, A, Mills, J, Mulhern, R and Short, N (2004) *Cognitive Behavioural Therapy in Mental Health Care.* London: Sage Publications.

Grant, A, Townend, M, Mills, J and Cockx, A (2008) *Assessment and Case Formulation in Cognitive Behavioural Therapy.* London: Sage Publications.

Greenberg, LS (2007) Emotion in the therapeutic relationship in emotion-focused therapy, in Gilbert, P and Leahy, R (eds) *The Therapeutic Relationship in the Cognitive Behavioural Psychotherapies.* Hove: Routledge.

Grover, SM (2005) Shaping effective communication skills and therapeutic relationships at work: the foundation of collaboration. *American Association of Occupational Health Nurses Journal*, 53: 177.

Hall, ET (1966) *The Hidden Dimension.* New York: Doubleday.

Hargie, O (ed.) (2006) *The Handbook of Communication Skills*, 3rd edition. London and New York: Routledge.

Hargie, O and Dickson, D (2004) *Skilled Interpersonal Communication. Research, Theory and Practice*, 4th edition. London and New York: Routledge.

Hartrick, G (1997) Relational capacity: the foundation for interpersonal nursing practice. *Journal of Advanced Nursing*, 26: 523–8.

Hayes, SC, Smith, S (2005) *Get Out of Your Mind and Into Your Life: The new acceptance and commitment therapy.* Oakland, CA: New Harbinger Publications.

Henderson, IW (1967) Psychological care of patients with malignant disease. *Applied Therapy*, 9(10): 827–32.

Hendricks, J and Hendricks, CD (1986) *Aging in Mass Society: Myths and realities*, 3rd edition. Boston, MA: Little, Brown.

Henley, A and Schott, J (1999) *Culture, Religion and Patient Care in a Multi-ethnic Society.* London: Age Concern.

Hewitt, JP (1998) *The Myth of Self-esteem: Finding happiness and solving problems in America.* New York: St Martin's Press.

Hofstede, G (1991) *Cultures and Organisation: The software of the mind.* London: McGraw-Hill.

Holstein, JA and Gubrium, JF (2000) *The Self We Live By: Narrative identity in a postmodern world.* New York and Oxford: Oxford University Press.

Honey, P and Mumford, A (1992) *The Manual of Learning Styles*, Maidenhead: Peter Honey Publications.

Howard, A (2001) Fallacies and realities of self. *Counselling and Psychotherapy Journal*, 12(4): 19–23.

Jasper, M (1996) The first year as a staff nurse: the experiences of a first cohort of Project 2000 nurses. *Journal of Advanced Nursing*, 24: 779–90.

Jones, A (2007) Putting practice into teaching: an exploratory study of nursing undergraduates' interpersonal skills and the effects of using empirical data as a teaching and learning resource. *Journal of Clinical Nursing*, 16: 2297–307.

Kagan, C, Evans, J and Kay, B (1986) *A Manual of Interpersonal Skills for Nurses: An experiential approach*. London: Harper and Row.

Kitson, AL (2003) A comparative analysis of lay-caring and professional (nursing) caring relationships. *International Journal of Nursing Studies*, 40(5): 503–10.

Kohut, H (1984) *How Does Analysis Cure?* Chicago, IL: University of Chicago Press.

Kolb, DA (2000) *Facilitators Guide to Learning*, Boston, MA: Hay/McBer.

Kolb, DA and Fry, D (1975) Towards an applied theory of experiential learning, in Cooper, CL (ed.) *Theories of Group Processes*. Chichester: Wiley.

Kreps, G and Kunimoto, EN (1994) *Effective Communication in Multicultural Health Care Settings*. London. Sage Publications.

Kyle, TV (1995) The concept of caring: a review of the literature. *Journal of Advanced Nursing*, 21: 506–14.

Lauder, W, Reynolds, W, Smith, A and Sharkey, S (2002) A comparison of therapeutic commitment, role support, role competency and empathy in three cohorts of nursing students. *Journal of Psychiatric and Mental Health Nursing*, 9: 483–91.

Lea, A, Watson, R and Deary, IJ (1998) Caring in nursing: a multivariate analysis. *Journal of Advanced Nursing*, 28: 662–71.

Leininger, MM (1978) *Transcultural Nursing*. New York: Wiley.

Leininger, MM (1981) The phenomenon of caring: importance, research questions and theoretical considerations, in Leininger, MM (ed.) *Caring, and Essential Human Need*. Detroit, MI: Wayne State University Press.

Leininger, MM (1984) *Care: The essence of nursing and health*. Detroit, MI: Wayne State University Press.

Leininger, MM (1997) Transcultural nursing research to nursing education and practice: 40 years. *Image: Journal of Nursing Scholarship*, 29(4): 341–7.

Long, A (ed.) (1989) *Interaction for Practice in Community Nursing*. Basingstoke: Macmillan.

Lovering, S (2006) Cultural attitudes and beliefs about pain. *Journal of Transcultural Nursing*, 17(4): 389–95.

Maben, JA, Latter, SB and Clark, JM (2006) The theory–practice gap: impact of professional-bureaucratic work conflict on newly-qualified nurses. *Journal of Advanced Nursing*, 55(4): 465–77.

Maben, JA, Latter, SB and Clark, JM (2007) The sustainability of ideals, values and the nursing mandate: evidence from a longitudinal qualitative study. *Nursing Inquiry*, 14: 99–113.

McCabe, C and Timmins, F (2006) *Communication Skills for Nursing Practice*, London: Palgrave Macmillan.

Macleod Clark, J (1985) The development of research in interpersonal skills, in Kagan, C (ed.) *Interpersonal Skills in Nursing: Research and applications*. London: Croom Helm, pp9–21.

McMahon, R (1993) Therapeutic nursing: theory, issues and practice, in McMahon, R and Pearson, A (eds) *Nursing as Therapy*, 2nd edition. London: Chapman Hall.

MacNaught, A (1994) A discriminating service: the socioeconomic and scientific roots of racial discrimination in the National Health Service. *Journal of Inter-Professional Care*, 8: 143–9.

Macpherson of Cluny, W (Chair) (1999) *The Stephen Lawrence Inquiry*. London: Stationery Office.

Maslin-Prothero, S (ed.) (2005) *Bailliere's Study Skills for Nurses and Midwives*, Oxford: Bailliere Tindall.

Melia, K (1984) Student nurses' construction of occupational socialisation. *Sociology of Health & Illness*, 2(2): 132–51.

Menzies Lyth, I (1988) *Containing Anxiety in Institutions: Selected essays*. London: Free Association Books.

Meyerson, DE (2002) If emotions were honoured: a cultural analysis, in Fineman, S (ed.) *Emotion in Organizations.* 2nd edition. London: Sage Publications.

Miranda, R and Andersen, SM (2007) The therapeutic relationship: implications from social cognition and transference, in Gilbert, P and Leahy, RL (eds) *The Therapeutic Relationship in the Cognitive Behavioural Psychotherapies.* Hove: Routledge.

Moon, J (2002) *How To Use Level Descriptors*. London: SEEC.

Morgan, G (1997*) Images of Organization*, 2nd edition. Thousand Oaks, CA: Sage Publications.

Morrison, P and Burnard, P (1991) *Caring and Communicating: The interpersonal relationship in nursing.* Basingstoke: Macmillan.

Morse, JM, Bottorff, J, Neander, W and Solberg, S (1991) Comparative analysis of conceptualisations and theories of caring. *Image: Journal of Nursing Scholarship*, 23(2): 119–26.

Morse, JM, Bottorff, J, Anderson, G, O'Brien, B and Solberg, S (1992) Beyond empathy: expanding expressing of caring. *Journal of Advanced Nursing*, 17: 809–21.

Muir Gray, JA (1997) *Evidence-based Healthcare: How to make health policy and management decisions.* New York: Churchill-Livingstone.

Mullen, CA (2005) *Mentorship Primer*, New York: Peter Lang.

Narayanasamy, A (2002) The ACCESS model: a transcultural nursing practice framework. *British Journal of Nursing*, 11(9): 643–50.

Narayanasamy, A and White, E (2005) A review of transcultural nursing. *Nurse Education Today*, 25: 102–11.

National Health Service Modernisation Agency (2003) *Essence of Care, Guidance and New Communication Benchmarks.* London: Department of Health.

Newell, R and Gournay, K (eds) (2000) *Mental Health Nursing. An evidence-based approach*. London: Churchill-Livingstone.

Nursing and Midwifery Council (NMC) (2004a) *Standards of Proficiency for Pre-registration Nursing Education*. London: NMC.

Nursing and Midwifery Council (NMC) (2004b) *The NMC Code of Professional Conduct: Standards for conduct, performance and ethics.* London: NMC.

Nursing and Midwifery Council (NMC) (2007) *Guidance for the Introduction of the Essential Skills Clusters for Pre-registration Nursing Programmes.* London: NMC.

Nussbaum, JF, Pecchioni, LL, Robinson, JD and Thompson, TL (2000) *Communication and Aging*, 2nd edition. Mahwah, NJ: Lawrence Erlbaum Associates.

Oakes, P, Haslam, A and Turner, J (1994) *Stereotypes and social reality.* Oxford: Blackwell.

Oliver, M (1990) *The Politics of Disablement.* London. Macmillan Press.

Padesky, C (1991) Schema as self-prejudice. Reprinted from the *International Cognitive Therapy Newsletter*, 6: 6–7 (1990). Copyright © 1991, Newport Beach, CA: Center for Cognitive Therapy.

Parfitt, B (1998) *Working Across Culture: A study of expatriate nurses working in developing countries in primary health care.* Aldershot: Ashage.

Peel, N (2003) Critical care: the role of the critical care nurse in the delivery of bad news. *British Journal of Nursing*, 12: 966–71.

Pender, NJ, Murdaugh, C and Parsons, MA (2006) *Health Promotion in Nursing Practice*, 5th edition. Upper Saddle River, NJ: Prentice-Hall Health.

Petrie, P (1997) *Communicating with Children and Adults: Interpersonal Skills for Early Years and Play Work.* London: Arnold.

Pfeffer, J (1981) *Power in Organizations.* Marshfield, MA: Pitman Publishing.

Platt, L (2005) *Migration and Social Mobility: The life chances of Britain's minority ethnic communities.* London: Joseph Rowntree Foundation.

Quinn, F and Hughes, S (2007) *Quinn's Principles and Practice of Nurse Education.* Oxford: Nelson Thornes.

Radsma, J (1994) Caring and nursing: a dilemma, *Journal of Advanced Nursing*, 20: 444–9.

Rees, C and Sheard, C (2004) Undergraduate medical students' views about a reflective portfolio assessment of their communication skills learning. *Medical Education*, 38: 125–8.

Reynolds, WJ and Scott, B (2000) Do nurses and other professional helpers normally display much empathy? Integrative literature reviews and meta-analyses. *Journal of Advanced Nursing*, 31(1): 226–34.

Robb, M and Douglas, J (2004) Managing diversity. *Nursing Management UK*, 11(1): 25–9.

Rodgers, BL and Cowles, KV (1997) A conceptual foundation for human suffering in nursing care and research. *Journal of Advanced Nursing*, 25: 1048–53.

Rogers, CR (1961) *On Becoming a Person.* Boston, MA: Houghton Mifflin.

Rogers, CR (1967) *On Becoming a Person: A therapist's view of psychotherapy.* London: Constable.

Rogers, CR (2002) *Client Centred Therapy.* London: Constable.

Rolfe, G, Freshwater, D and Jasper, M (2001) *Critical Reflection for Nursing and the Helping Professions: A users' guide.* Basingstoke: Palgrave.

Rose, D and Pevalin, DJ (2005) *The National Statistics Socio-economic Classification: Origins, development and use.* Institute for Social and Economic Research, University of Essex. Basingstoke: Palgrave Macmillan.

Ruesch, J (1961) *Therapeutic Communication.* Toronto: Norton.

Ryan, EB and Hamilton, JM (1994) Patronizing the old: how do younger and older adults respond to baby talk in the nursing home? *International Journal of Aging and Human Development*, 39(1): 21–32.

Sapir, E (ed. Mandelbaum, DG) (1983) *Selected writings of Edward Sapir in Language, Culture and Personality*. Berkeley, CA: University of California Press.

Sawley, L (2001) Perceptions of racism in the Health Service. *Nursing Standard*, 24 January, 15(19): 33–5.

Siviter, B and Stevens, D (2004) *The Student Nurse Handbook: A survival guide*. Oxford: Bailliere Tindall.

Sloane, J (1992) Offences and defences against patients: a psychoanalytical view of the borderline between empathic failure and malpractice. *Canadian Journal of Psychology*, 38: 265–73.

Smith, A (1997) Learning about reflection. *Journal of Advanced Nursing*, 28: 891–8.

Smith, A and Jack, K (2005) Reflective practice: a meaningful task for students. *Nursing Standard*, 19: 33–7.

Smith, CE (1987) *Patient Education: Nurses in partnership with other health professionals.* Orlando, FL: Grune & Stratton.

Spichiger, E, Walhagen, MI and Benner, P (2005) Nursing as a caring practice. *Scandinavian Journal of Caring Science*, 19: 303–9.

Stokes, G (1991) A transcultural nurse is about. *Senior Nurse*, 11(1): 40–2.

Tait, A (1985) Interpersonal skill issues arising from mastectomy contexts, in Kagan, C (ed.) *Interpersonal Skills in Nursing: Research and applications*. London: Croom-Helm, pp165–84.

Taylor, J (2003) *Foundations in Nursing and Health Care: Study skills in health care.* Cheltenham: Nelson Thornes.

Teekman, B (2000) Exploring reflective practice in nursing. *Journal of Advanced Nursing*, 31: 1125–35.

Thompson, D (ed.) (1995) *The Concise Oxford Dictionary of Current English*, 9th edition. Oxford: Clarendon Press.

Thompson, N (2001) *Anti-discriminatory Practice*, 3rd edition. Basingstoke: Palgrave Macmillan.

Thwaites, R and Bennett-Levy, J (2007) Conceptualizing empathy in cognitive behaviour therapy: making the implicit explicit. In press for *Behavioural and Cognitive Psychotherapy.*

Timmins, F (2007) Communication skills: revisiting the fundamentals. *Nurse Prescribing*, 5: 395–9.

Trinder, L and Reynolds, S (eds) (2000) *Evidence-based Practice: A critical appraisal*. Oxford: Blackwell.

Watson, J (1988) *Nursing: Human science and human care*, 3rd edition. New York: National League for Nursing.

Watson, J and Foster, R (2003) The attending nurse caring model: integrating theory, evidence and advanced caring-healing therapeutics for transforming professional practice, *Journal of Clinical Nursing*, 12(3): 360–5.

Whitton, E (2003) *Humanistic Approach to Psychotherapy*. Chichester: Wiley Blackwell.

Whorf, B (ed. Carroll, J) (1956) *Language, Thought and Reality: Selected writings of Benjamin Lee Whorf*. Boston, MA: MIT Press.

Wilkins, H (1993) Transcultural nursing: a selective review of the literature, 1985–1991. *Journal of Advanced Nursing*, 18: 602–16.

World Health Organization (2000) *World Health Report 2000 – Health Systems: Improving performance*. Geneva: WHO.

Wurzbach, ME (1999) The moral metaphors of nursing. *Journal of Advanced Nursing*. 30(1): 94–9.

Wyer, RS and Srull, TK (1986) Human cognition in its social context. *Psychological Review*, 93: 322–59.

Index